GLAUCOMA SURGERY

GLAUCOMA SURGERY

S. FABIÁN LERNER, M.D.

Director
Glaucoma Section
Postgraduate Department
University Favaloro School of Medicine
Buenos Aires, Argentina

RICHARD K. PARRISH II, M.D.

Professor
Associate Dean for Graduate Medical Education
Department of Ophthalmology
University of Miami School of Medicine
Chairman
Graduate Medical Education Committee
Jackson Memorial Hospital
Jackson Health System
Miami, Florida

Illustrations by Haroldo Ruquet

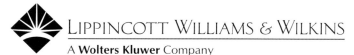

LIPPINCOTT WILLIAMS & WILKINS
A **Wolters Kluwer** Company
Philadelphia · Baltimore · New York · London
Buenos Aires · Hong Kong · Sydney · Tokyo

Acquisitions Editor: Jonathan Pine
Developmental Editor: Joanne Bersin
Production Editor: Jodi Borgenicht
Manufacturing Manager: Benjamin Rivera
Cover Designer: Jeane Norton
Compositor: Lippincott Williams & Wilkins Desktop Division
Printer: Walsworth Publishing Co.

Library of Congress Cataloging-in-Publication Data

Lerner, S. Fabián.
   [Cirugía de glaucoma. English]
   Glaucoma surgery / S. Fabián Lerner, Richard K. Parrish II.
      p. ; cm.
   Includes bibliographical references and index.
   Translated from Spanish.
   ISBN 0-7817-3732-X
   1. Glaucoma—Surgery. I. Parrish, Richard K. II. Title.
   [DNLM: 1. Glaucoma—surgery. WW 290 L6165c 2003]
   RE871 .L4213 2003
   617.7′41059—dc21

                                    2002043055

Care has been taken to confirm the accuracy of the information presented and to describe generally accepted practices. However, the authors and publisher are not responsible for errors or omissions or for any consequences from application of the information in this book and make no warranty, expressed or implied, with respect to the currency, completeness, or accuracy of the contents of the publication. Application of this information in a particular situation remains the professional responsibility of the practitioner.

The authors and publisher have exerted every effort to ensure that drug selection and dosage set forth in this text are in accordance with current recommendations and practice at the time of publication. However, in view of ongoing research, changes in government regulations, and the constant flow of information relating to drug therapy and drug reactions, the reader is urged to check the package insert for each drug for any change in indications and dosage and for added warnings and precautions. This is particularly important when the recommended agent is a new or infrequently employed drug.

Some drugs and medical devices presented in this publication have Food and Drug Administration (FDA) clearance for limited use in restricted research settings. It is the responsibility of the health care provider to ascertain the FDA status of each drug or device planned for use in their clinical practice.

10 9 8 7 6 5 4 3 2 1

CONTENTS

GLAUCOMA SURGERY

INDICATIONS, PREOPERATIVE EVALUATION, AND ANESTHESIA

The purpose of glaucoma treatment is to maintain visual function and prevent further loss. Although many factors may contribute to glaucomatous optic neuropathy, reduction of intraocular pressure (IOP) remains the primary therapeutic goal. Medical treatment and laser or incisional surgery to lower IOP prevents additional visual field loss in most patients with primary open-angle glaucoma (1,2). The detailed discussion of the preoperative assessment, surgical technique, and postoperative care of patients with glaucoma is the focus of this book.

INDICATIONS

Glaucoma filtering surgery, such as trabeculectomy, is performed when medical treatment or laser therapy or both fails to reduce IOP from a level that has been associated with progressive visual field loss or optic nerve damage. Ineffectiveness, intolerance, and poor compliance with medical therapy support the decision for surgical intervention (3).

PREOPERATIVE EVALUATION

Several important aspects should be considered when assessing the risks and benefits of glaucoma filtering surgery.

Patient Age and Life Expectancy

Patients younger than 50 years old may heal more vigorously after filtering surgery than older patients and have poorer prognoses unless medications that modify wound healing, such as mitomycin C (MMC) or 5-fluorouracil (5-FU), are used (4). In view of their longer life expectancy, younger patients are also at greater risk for visual loss. The cumulative long-term risks of complications, such as bleb leaks, bleb infections, and endophthalmitis, are also higher, particularly when antimetabolites are used.

General Health Status

Although glaucoma filtering surgery risks are usually limited to those of local anesthetics and ocular complications, knowledge of general medical conditions, such as diabetes, hypertension, cardiac status, and anticoagulant use, is important. What medications does the patient usually take? Specifically, patients should be asked if they take aspirin, vitamin E, or gingko biloba extracts, since many do not consider these over-the-counter preparations as "medications." Such medications should be discontinued 3 to 4 weeks preoperatively, as they may increase the risk of intraoperative or postoperative hemorrhage. The value of routine laboratory examinations, such as complete blood count, urinalysis, or serum electrolytes, has not been demonstrated in patients undergoing cataract surgery. The general medical history and examination should guide the decision to order preoperative studies for glaucoma patients.

Disease Duration

How long has the patient taken topical medications? Evidence suggests that prolonged topical therapy, particularly with α-adrenergic medications and miotics, may induce inflammatory cells in the subconjunctival space and predispose to filtering surgery failure (5,6).

Intraocular Pressure

Although very high IOP associated with decreased optic nerve perfusion, intermittent visual obscurations, and central retinal artery pulsations must be lowered right away, usually filtering surgery is more safely performed after the initiation of medical treatment. The risk of postoperative or delayed suprachoroidal hemorrhage after filtering surgery is greatest in eyes with very high preoperative IOP and may be reduced by lowering IOP prior to surgery (7). If the IOP is greater than 35 mm Hg, an intravenous hyperosmotic agent may be given. Mannitol 20% solution, the most commonly used intravenous agent, is given at a dose of 0.5 to 1 mg/kg at least 1 hour before surgery over a period of 30 to 40 minutes. Extreme caution should be taken when administering this agent to patients with cardiovascular or renal disease, such as congestive heart failure or chronic renal failure. Medical consultation should be sought before recommending their use in these patients. For patients who cannot safely receive hyperosmotic agents, a 27- or 30-gauge needle or needle knife paracentesis tract permits gradual and controlled IOP reduction.

Optic Nerve and Visual Field Status

The extent of the optic nerve damage, visual field loss, and the rate of progression are important factors to consider when planning surgical intervention. Assessment of optic nerve status with stereoscopic photographs or computerized disc studies and review of serial visual fields provide insight into the rapidity of the disease course. In eyes with advanced disc or rapid visual field loss, the recommendation for surgery is made earlier. Eyes with advanced glaucomatous optic neuropathy may also require very low IOP (10 to 12 mm Hg) to minimize further progression (8).

Visual Acuity and Refractive Error

Management of the patient's expectations regarding visual acuity is an important part of the preoperative informed consent process. The surgeon should warn the patient that postoperative visual acuity might diminish in the immediate postoperative period but usually returns to the preoperative level within a few weeks. Sudden loss of central vision immediately after surgery ("snuff-out") is an uncommon, but real, concern to patient and surgeon alike. The risk is probably less than the 13.6% reported, and those with central visual field loss immediately adjacent to the point of fixation seem to be most vulnerable (9). The patient and family members must clearly understand that the primary goal of filtering surgery is to lower IOP and preserve visual function rather than to improve central visual acuity, as in cataract surgery. The importance of frequent postoperative examinations should also be understood. Preoperative knowledge of the anticipated blurring of vision and the need for frequent visits will alleviate postoperative anxiety. The long-term risk of vision loss as a result of uncontrolled glaucoma should be put in perspective (10).

Other Ocular Conditions

Visually significant cataract and uncontrolled IOP argue for a combined cataract extraction–trabeculectomy procedure rather than trabeculectomy alone. The decision making process and technical aspects of combined cataract–glaucoma operation are discussed in Chapter 11. Trabeculectomy, even when uncomplicated and not associated with hypotony or flat anterior chamber, may accelerate cataract progression. If previous filtering surgery has been performed, usually conjunctival scarring is present at the original filtering site. In the preoperative slit-lamp examination, attempting to move the conjunctiva overlying the filtering site with a cotton-tipped applicator moistened with tetracaine hydrochloride ophthalmic solution USP 0.5% may allow assessment of the extent of scarring. If the conjunctiva is not moveable, filtering surgery at another site or drainage implant surgery may be considered. The use of medications to modify wound healing in these patients is discussed in Chapter 9.

External Diseases

The ocular surface should be examined for infectious blepharitis or conjunctivitis, decreased tear production, and subconjunctival scarring. The nasolacrimal sac should be compressed and the inferior punctum examined for purulent exudation associated with dacryocystitis. Culture for microorganisms should be performed as indicated by the severity of the condition. Punctate epithelial erosions associated with keratoconjunctivitis sicca should be vigorously managed preoperatively with a nonpreserved tear substitute. Postoperative subconjunctival 5-FU injections may worsen corneal epitheliopathy and predispose to the formation of frank corneal epithelial defects. Some corneal epithelial irregularities are associated with subconjunctival scarring, misdirected lash growth, shortening of the inferior cul de sac, and symblepharon formation. This condition, termed pseudopemphigoid or drug-induced conjunctival scarring, has been associated with topical glaucoma medications, usually strong miotics, and resembles ocular cicatricial pemphigoid (11,12) (Figs. 1.1 and 1.2).

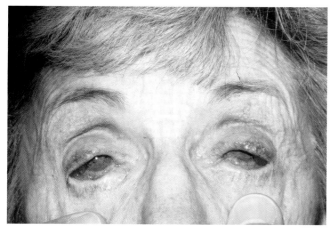

FIGURE 1.1. Bilateral conjunctival scarring associated with chronic phospholine iodide use (pseudopemphigoid). (Reprinted from Parrish RK II, ed. *University of Miami Bascom Palmer Eye Institute Atlas of Ophthalmology.* Philadelphia: Current Medicine, 2000:218, with permission.)

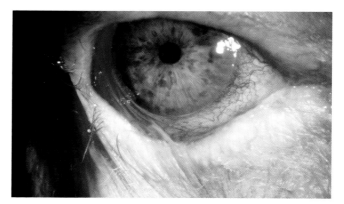

FIGURE 1.2. Drug-induced conjunctival scarring. Note shortening of inferior conjunctival cul de sac and inferior symblepharon. (Reprinted from Parrish RK II, ed. *University of Miami Bascom Palmer Eye Institute Atlas of Ophthalmology.* Philadelphia: Current Medicine, 2000:218, with permission.)

The Contralateral Eye

The outcome of filtering surgery in the fellow eye may predict the postoperative course of the second eye. If both eyes require filtering surgery, we prefer operating on the eye with the lower visual potential first. The possibility of serious complication, such as suprachoroidal hemorrhage, excessive filtration, or flat anterior chamber, in the eye with poorer acuity may guide the surgeon in planning intervention in the second eye. However, this generalization does not preclude the possibility of operating on the eye with the better potential acuity first, if the IOP is very high or the rate of visual field loss is accelerated.

Surgical Prognosis

Some types of glaucoma in eyes with poorer than usual prognoses, such as after cataract surgery, previous failed filtering surgery, or with chronic intraocular inflammation, and in younger patients or African American or Caribbean patients, argue for the application of 5-FU or MMC in addition to trabeculectomy (see Chapter 9) or implantation of a glaucoma drainage device (see Chapter 12) or cyclodestruction (see Chapter 15).

Preoperative Ocular Medications

Cholinesterase inhibitors, such as Phospholine iodide (echothiophate) and Humorsol (demecarium bromide), which also inhibit pseudocholinesterase, should be discontinued 2 weeks before surgery. Use of these drugs in patients who receive succinylcholine during intubation for general anesthesia may lead to prolonged apnea, and the anesthesiologist should be aware of this history. Miotics, such as pilocarpine hydrochloride, may promote postoperative inflammation and breakdown of the blood aqueous barrier and should be discontinued 2 or 3 days before surgery. However, 4% pilocarpine hydrochloride instilled 2 hours before the procedure maintains pupillary miosis after retrobulbar or peribulbar anesthesia and minimizes iris prolapse. Although the value of preoperative prophylactic topical antibiotics has not been demonstrated, some surgeons recommend the application of a combination antibiotic–steroid drop for 2 or 3 days before surgery. This may provide an anti-inflammatory effect and reduce the microbial population, but is unlikely to contribute to the selective overgrowth of antibiotic-resistant organisms.

Anesthesia

Glaucoma filtering surgery is usually performed in most cooperative adults under local (retrobulbar, peribulbar, sub-Tenon's, or topical) and in children under general anesthesia. For peribulbar or retrobulbar anesthesia, 2% lidocaine hydrochloride without epinephrine or 0.75% bupivacaine hydrochloride is effective. We do not recommend using ocular compression with a Honan balloon to assist in the distribution of the anesthetic within the orbit as this could alter blood flow to a glaucomatous optic nerve. In a cooperative patient, sub-Tenon's or topical anesthesia (2% lidocaine as Xylocaine 2% jelly, AstraZeneca LP, Wilmington, DE) is preferred by many surgeons. Under topical anesthesia, cauterization of the episcleral surface and completion of the peripheral iridectomy may produce pain. If needed, approximately 0.1 mL of nonpreserved lidocaine (1.0% Xylocaine-MPF, AstraZeneca LP, Wilmington, DE) can be injected into the anterior chamber to minimize discomfort during combined cataract and glaucoma procedures.

REFERENCES

1. Sherwood MB, Migdal CS, Hitchings RA, et al. Initial treatment of glaucoma: surgery or medications. *Surv Ophthalmol* 1993;37:293–305.
2. Lichter PR, Musch DC, Gillespie BW, et al. Interim clinical outcomes in the Collaborative Initial

Glaucoma Treatment Study comparing initial treatment randomized to medications or surgery. *Ophthalmology* 2001;108:1943–1953.

3. Katz JL, Costa VP, Spaeth GL. Filtration surgery. In: Ritch R, Shields MB, Krupin T, eds. *The glaucomas.* St. Louis: Mosby, 1996:1662–1664.

4. Gressel MG, Heuer DK, Parrish RK II. Trabeculectomy in young patients. *Ophthalmology* 1984;91:1242–1246.

5. Johnson DH, Yoshikawa K, Brubaker RF, et al. The effect of long-term medical therapy on the outcome of filtration surgery. *Am J Ophthalmol* 1994;117:139–148.

6. Lavin MJ, Wormald RP, Migdal CS, et al. The influence of prior therapy on the success of trabeculectomy. *Arch Ophthalmol* 1990;108:1543–1548.

7. The Fluorouracil Filtering Surgery Study Group. Risk factors for suprachoroidal hemorrhage after filtering surgery. *Am J Ophthalmol* 1992;113:501–507.

8. The AGIS Investigators. The Advanced Glaucoma Intervention Study (AGIS): 7. The relationship between control of intraocular pressure and visual field deterioration. *Am J Ophthalmol* 2000;130: 429–440.

9. Kolker AE. Visual prognosis in advanced glaucoma: a comparison of medical and surgical therapy for retention of vision in 101 eyes with advanced glaucoma. *Trans Am Ophthalmol Soc* 1977;75: 539–555.

10. Costa VP, Smith M, Spaeth GL, et al. Loss of visual acuity after trabeculectomy. *Ophthalmology* 1993;100:599–612.

11. Patten JT, Cavanagh HD, Allansmith MR. Induced ocular pseudopemphigoid. *Am J Ophthalmol* 1976;82:272–276.

12. Pouliquen Y, Patey A, Foster CS, et al. Drug-induced cicatricial pemphigoid affecting the conjunctiva; light and electron microscopic features. *Ophthalmology* 1986;93:775–782.

ANATOMY FOR
THE GLAUCOMA SURGEON

Corneal–scleral or limbal anatomy should be thoroughly understood by anyone performing glaucoma surgery. The surgical limbus is a blue–gray transition zone between the parallel collagen fibers of the peripheral cornea and those of the anterior sclera. The anterior border is coincident with an imaginary vertical line between the peripheral edge of Bowman's and Descemet's membranes. The posterior border, covered by overlying conjunctiva and Tenon's capsule, is defined by the transition between the white scleral tissue and the blue–gray zone. The limbus, widest superiorly at the 12:00 meridian, measures 1.0 to 1.5 mm and progressively becomes narrower inferiorly, nasally, and temporally (1–4) (Fig. 2.1).

The conjunctiva, a mobile vascularized tissue with a surface epithelium, inserts in the peripheral corneal epithelium at the anterior limbal edge. Tenon's capsule, a loose fibrovascular layer, attaches approximately 1.5 to 2.0 mm posterior to the conjunctival insertion. This capsule, usually thicker and more vascular in young patients, is firmly attached at the 10:30 and 1:30 meridians. In standard trabeculectomy with either a fornix-based or limbus-based flap, both the conjunctiva and Tenon's capsule are incised and dissected to expose the underlying sclera and limbus. In a limbus-based conjunctival flap, the conjunctival insertion defines the anterior limit of the dissection. The posterior border incision of the scleral flap should begin peripheral to the gray–white scleral tissue. As the dissection advances, a relatively bright curvilinear white line parallel to the limbus is exposed that corresponds to the scleral spur. Proceeding anterior to the scleral spur, the bed of the flap appears darker and more transparent. This zone, immediately anterior to scleral spur, corresponds to the underlying trabecular meshwork and Schlemm's canal. Specifically, Schlemm's canal is located in the most posterior area of the blue–gray limbus, immediately anterior to the sclerolimbal border. This very important anatomic landmark guides the surgeon when identifying Schlemm's canal for trabeculotomy or viscocanalostomy. In dissecting forward, the angulation of the blade should be changed to follow the limbal curvature and to avoid premature entry into the anterior chamber. The union between the sclera and the cornea forms a visible change in limbal curvature, the external scleral sulcus, which is the junction of the two different radii of curvature. The internal scleral sulcus corresponds to the internal part of the limbus that holds the trabecular meshwork, and in its posterior and lateral zone lays Schlemm's canal.

The dissection of the scleral flap should continue into clear cornea, anterior to Schwalbe's line. This is the point where entry is made into the anterior chamber (see Chapter 5). The transition between the white sclera and the blue–gray limbus is posteriorly displaced at the deepest point of the scleral bed in comparison with its position at the scleral surface. The oblique insertion of the peripheral corneal fibers into the sclera may create the impression that the flap dissection was sufficiently anterior and led to premature entry into the anterior chamber, more posteriorly than desired. *Scleral flap dissection should be continued anteriorly until clear cornea is encountered.* The posterior or scleral border of the inner block should be placed anteriorly to the scleral spur. Cutting or excising scleral tissue posterior to the scleral spur carries the risk of damaging the ciliary body and major circle of the iris and causing intraocular bleeding (see Chapters 5 and 7). The nor-

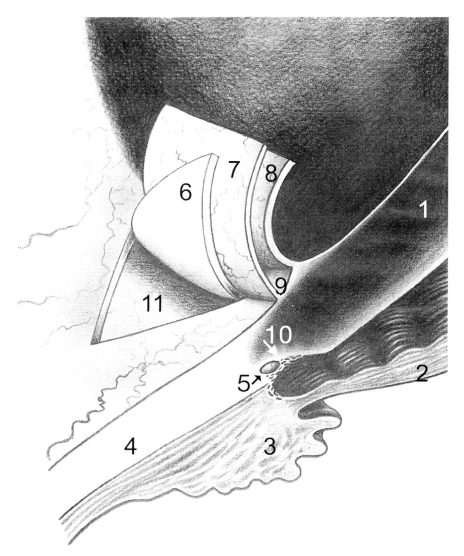

FIGURE 2.1. Limbal anatomy. 1, cornea; 2, iris; 3, ciliary body; 4, sclera; 5, Schlemm's canal; 6, scleral flap; 7, Tenon's capsule; 8, conjunctiva; 9, external scleral sulcus; 10, internal scleral sulcus; 11, sclera–limbus junction.

mal anatomic landmarks in adult eyes with glaucoma may be substantially altered in babies and children, especially in buphthalmic eyes with primary infantile glaucoma, where the sclera is much thinner than usual. The limbal tissue stretches in response to the elevated intraocular pressure (IOP), and the posterior scleral–corneal border appears more peripheral than in adults.

Underlying the sclera, just posterior to the scleral spur, is the pars plicata of the ciliary body that terminates in the pars plana, approximately 2.5 to 3.5 mm posterior to the limbus. Hemorrhage may occur if the surgeon injures the ciliary body or major circle of the iris when removing the inner scleral block or performing the peripheral iridectomy. Iridectomy does not usually cause bleeding; however, iris neovascularization and chronic inflammation predispose to oozing. Usually irrigation of the anterior chamber with balanced salt solution (BSS) or direct compression of the iris root with a cellulose sponge results in prompt hemostasis. In these eyes, viscoelastics introduced through the paracentesis tract may be used to tamponade the bleeding vessels.

Two long anterior ciliary arteries run forward in each rectus muscle, except the lateral rectus, which has only one. In addition to these arteries and associated veins, perforating

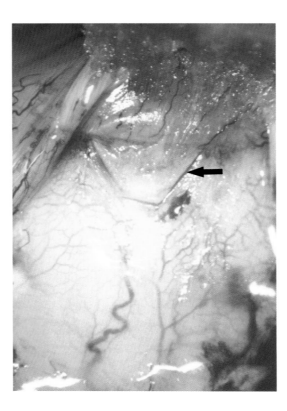

FIGURE 2.2. Scleral flap position anterior to perforating vessels (*arrow*).

scleral blood vessels (neurovascular loops of Axenfeld) are often encountered when dissecting the scleral flap. *The surgeon should position the trabeculectomy flap in an area without perforating vessels to minimize bleeding* (Fig 2.2). The oozing from episcleral or scleral vessels in patients taking antiglaucoma medications for the long term, especially miotics and adrenergic agonists, may interfere with visualization and contribute to postoperative wound healing. Light cauterization to minimize hemorrhage should be applied only to the bleeding vessel, but the scleral flap should not be treated so as to avoid tissue shrinkage. Scleral flap shrinkage may complicate closure by not permitting adjustment of sutures to the proper tension for the desired rate of aqueous humor flow. Particular care should be taken to avoid cauterizing the conjunctival incision, which may cause early wound leakage.

SURGICAL PEARLS

- Select the 12:00 meridian for the trabeculectomy flap. The limbus is widest superiorly and becomes progressively narrower inferiorly, nasally, and temporally.
- Avoid trabeculectomy in the inferior limbus. Inferiorly located filtering blebs are at high risk for developing blebitis and endophthalmitis.
- Avoid perforating vessels (neurovascular loops of Axenfeld) that penetrate the sclera and are associated with episcleral pigmentation.
- Confirm that the scleral flap dissection extends into peripheral clear cornea before entering the anterior chamber. Remember that the junction of the sclera and the blue–gray limbus is more posteriorly displaced at the depth of the scleral bed than the scleral surface.
- Position the posterior border of the scleral excision or inner block anterior to the scleral spur. Failure to do so may result in inadvertent injury to the ciliary body or blood vessels within the major circle of the iris.

REFERENCES

1. Hogan MJ, Alvarado JA, Wedell JE. The limbus. In: Hogan MJ, Alvarado JA, Weddell JE, eds. *Histology of the human eye;* an atlas and textbook. Philadelphia: WB Saunders, 1971:112–182.
2. Minckler DS: Anatomy and glaucoma surgery. In: Weinreb RN, Mills RP, eds. *Glaucoma surgery: principles and techniques*, 2nd ed. San Francisco: American Academy of Ophthalmology, 1998:8–17.
3. Minckler DS. Anatomy in glaucoma-related surgery. In: Waltman SR, Keates RH, Hoyt CS, et al., eds. *Surgery of the eye*. New York: Churchill Livingstone,1988;1:311–322.
4. Shields MB. *Textbook of glaucoma*, 4th ed. Philadelphia: Lippincott Williams & Wilkins, 2000: 456–460.

3

GONIOTOMY, STANDARD TRABECULOTOMY, AND MODIFIED TRABECULOTOMY

INDICATIONS

Goniotomy (*trabeculotomy ab interno*) and trabeculotomy (*trabeculotomy ab externo*) are usually performed for the surgical management of primary infantile glaucoma. In both procedures, the surgeon establishes a communication between Schlemm's canal and the anterior chamber (1). The likelihood of successful surgery is highest in primary infantile or congenital glaucoma and lower in glaucoma associated with developmental angle anomalies, such as aniridia or Rieger's syndrome.

When performing goniotomy, the incompletely developed trabecular meshwork is incised with a sharp needle or knife. In trabeculotomy, the inner wall of Schlemm's canal and trabecular meshwork are ruptured with a blunt-tipped probe (trabeculotome). To safely perform goniotomy, the surgeon must have a clear view of the anterior chamber angle. Goniotomy does not involve a conjunctiva incision or produce limbal scarring that could affect the outcome of future filtering procedures, such as trabeculectomy. Trabeculotomy may be performed in eyes with corneal edema that preclude clear visualization of the angle; however, limbal and scleral incisions may cause scarring. Although trabeculotomy has also been performed in adult glaucoma patients, the success rate is much lower than in primary infantile glaucoma.

Preoperatively, the parents should clearly understand the purpose of the examination under anesthesia and possible operation, including the risks and benefits of the intervention, the necessity for frequent postoperative visits to monitor intraocular pressure (IOP) and optic nerve status, and amblyopia management. Parents, deeply involved in the success of pediatric glaucoma surgery, should understand the complex nature of managing a condition that spans childhood and adolescence.

Every child with suspected primary infantile glaucoma should undergo a complete ocular examination prior to decision making regarding surgical intervention. Usually this examination is performed under general inhalation anesthesia and includes, in order of evaluation, tonometry [Perkins Hand Held Applanation Tonometer MK2 (Haag-Streit Ag, Közig, Switzerland); Tono-Pen XL Applanation Tonometer Product Number 23-0635 (Medtronic Ophthalmics, Jacksonville, FL; and Pneumotonometer Product Number 23-2340, Medtronic Ophthalmics, Jacksonville, FL)], anterior segment examination with an operating microscope or hand-held biomicroscope, gonioscopy, measurement of horizontal corneal diameters, axial length determination with A-scan echography, and examination of the optic disc. Most general inhalation agents, such as halothane (Fluothane), reduce IOP. Although some surgeons prefer measuring IOP as soon as stage I anesthesia is reached before intubation, several confounding factors may affect the accuracy of the IOP determination at this level, such as pressure of the mask against the orbit and Valsalva maneuvers. Establishment of a patent and reliable airway is a primary concern for patient safety. As soon as a decision is reached regarding surgery, an endotracheal airway should be established and the child placed under general inhalation anesthesia.

GONIOTOMY

To perform this procedure successfully, the surgeon must have a clear view of the angle structures (2). To reduce corneal epithelial edema, oral acetazolamide may be given preoperatively at a recommended dose of 5 to 10 mg/kg of body weight every 4 to 6 hours. *Brimonidine (Alphagan or Alphagan P, Allergan, Irvine, CA) should not be used in children to reduce IOP as it can cause respiratory depression and apnea.* If preoperative acetazolamide does not clear corneal edema, the surgeon may remove the cloudy central epithelium by rubbing with a cotton applicator or a rounded blade. Care should be taken not to damage Bowman's membrane. In buphthalmic eyes, breaks in Descemet's membrane (Haab striae) and stromal edema may prevent clear visualization of the angle structures and do not clear with topical glycerin. If the angle structures are not seen, trabeculotomy or drainage implant surgery should be performed. After the optic nerve has been examined, one drop of 2% pilocarpine hydrochloride may be instilled to produce miosis and protect the lens.

Goniotomy is usually performed in the nasal angle with the surgeon seated at the temporal side of the patient. A goniotomy lens, such as the Barkan lens or the Swan-Jacob gonioprism (Ocular Instruments, Bellevue, WA), is used to view the angle. The Swan-Jacob gonioprism allows the surgeon to observe the angle without tilting the microscope by moving the handle of the lens (Fig 3.1). The goniotomy knife, such as the Barraquer or the Swan knife, or a 25-gauge needle on a tuberculin syringe may be used to incise the trabecular meshwork. The syringe filled with sterile balanced salt solution (BSS) or viscoelastic material is used to maintain anterior chamber depth during the procedure.

The assistant should be thoroughly familiar with every step of the procedure. He will be asked by the surgeon to rotate the globe to improve the view and maximize the extent

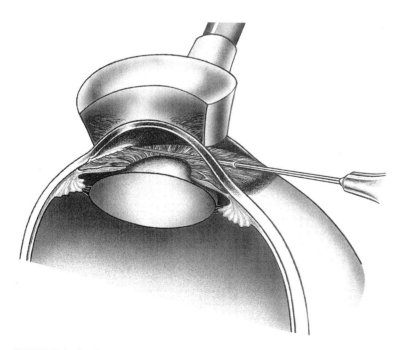

FIGURE 3.1. Gonioscopy. Swan-Jacob surgical goniolens and 25-gauge needle on a tuberculin syringe to incise angle structures.

of the angle treated. With nasal angle surgery, the assistant, seated at the head of the patient, grasps the insertion of the superior and inferior rectus muscles with two locking toothed forceps, such as the Castroviejo 0.5-mm forceps. If the goniotomy is performed in the inferior angle, the knife enters through the superior peripheral cornea and the assistant, seated at the temporal side of the patient, grasps the insertions of lateral and medial rectus muscles to rotate the globe. After positioning the gonioprism, the surgeon introduces the goniotomy knife or 25-gauge needle through the peripheral cornea just anterior to the limbus. The knife should be introduced obliquely to assure a watertight incision. The tip is advanced to the nasal angle, parallel to the plane of the iris, under direct visualization to avoid striking the lens, the cornea, or the iris. Alternatively, the knife or needle entry may be made after the anterior chamber has been filled with a viscoelastic material to maintain depth and the goniotomy lens has been placed on the eye. With the knife or needle under gonioscopic visualization, the surgeon cuts through the anterior trabecular meshwork for 4 to 6 clock hours (120 to 180 degrees) (Fig. 3.1). The knife should move smoothly with minimal resistance. If the knife sticks, the tip is probably positioned too deeply and is likely cutting through scleral fibers. As the incision of the trabecular meshwork continues, the iris retracts posteriorly and the peripheral anterior chamber deepens. After completion, the anterior chamber should be filled with either sterile balanced saline or viscoelastic material. Occasionally the surgeon encounters mild bleeding when the knife is withdrawn from the anterior chamber and the IOP drops acutely. Introduction of viscoelastic material at the beginning of the procedure may minimize this complication. The self-sealing peripheral clear corneal wound usually does not require sutures. A broad-spectrum antibiotic, such as ceftazidime (100 mg/mL), is usually given as a subconjunctival injection. Cycloplegic agents are not used.

TRABECULOTOMY

After placing a superior clear corneal traction suture, the surgeon dissects a fornix-based or a limbus-based conjunctival flap to expose the superior limbus. Light cautery with a battery-powered unit or bipolar diathermy controls bleeding from scleral vessels. Care should be taken to avoid excessive cautery that may shrink scleral tissue and alter limbal anatomy. The surgeon should dissect a thick scleral flap at approximately 80% depth anteriorly into the peripheral clear cornea to facilitate identification of Schlemm's canal. This is particularly helpful in buphthalmic eyes with distorted limbal anatomy. A 3-mm radial incision in the middle of the scleral flap identifies the tissue overlying Schlemm's canal (Fig. 3.2). The key anatomic landmark is the band of circumferential white fibers located in the depth of the scleral flap bed that corresponds to the scleral spur. Schlemm's canal is located immediately anterior to the scleral spur. The surgeon slowly cuts this tissue with a sharp instrument, such as a razor blade fragment, until perforating the external wall of Schlemm's canal. Upon entering the canal, aqueous humor or occasionally blood percolates through the incision. To confirm localization of the canal, the surgeon passes a 5-0 or 6-0 nylon suture, whose tip has been rounded by heating with a cautery unit, into both cut ends of the canal to a length of 2 or 3 clock hours (Fig. 3.3). Minimal resistance may be encountered in buphthalmic eyes; however, if the suture does not pass smoothly, it probably is not in the canal. Following withdrawal of the suture, a trabeculotome (right- or left-handed trabeculotome) is placed into one side of the canal. Some surgeons perform a paracentesis before introducing the trabeculotome if the anterior chamber requires reformation. Use of the double-armed Harms trabeculotome permits the surgeon to estimate the location of the internal blade within Schlemm's canal by observing the position of the arm outside the eye. After introducing the first trabeculotome in the anterior chamber, the eye may soften and make passage of the second trabeculotome more difficult. If the surgeon is right-hand dominant, it may be easier to introduce the trabeculotome into the right side first as this maneuver is usually performed with the left hand. The left side of the procedure is completed with the right hand more

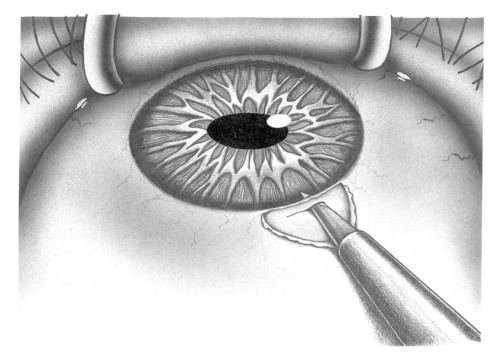

FIGURE 4.1. Beveled limbal incision.

iris prolapse. Inadvertent iris perforation at the time of anterior chamber entry and previous intraocular inflammation associated with extensive posterior synechiae may prevent prolapse. In this situation, the surgeon carefully grasps the peripheral iris and gently retracts it from the lips of the incision. Attention should be paid to grasping only the superficial iris stroma to avoid injury to the underlying anterior lens capsule. Only the portion of the iris that extends through the wound that is external to the incision should be cut with a Vannas or de Wecker scissors (Storz Instruments, Bausch & Lomb, Rochester, NY) held at the level of the superficial sclera. The position of the scissors and the amount of iris tissue removed determines the iridectomy shape. To produce a wide-based iridectomy with a rounded anterior edge, the scissors should be held parallel or tan-

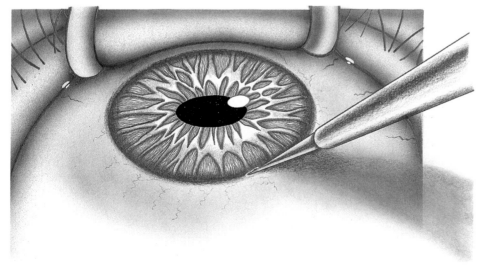

FIGURE 4.2. Clear corneal incision.

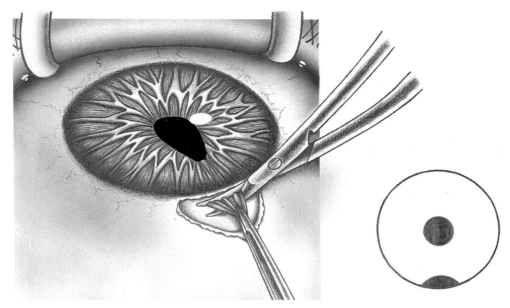

FIGURE 4.3. Peripheral iridectomy. A scissors held parallel to the limbus produces a broad basal iridectomy with a round contour (*inset*).

gent to the limbus (Fig. 4.3). If a narrower iridectomy with a triangular shape is chosen, the scissors should be oriented perpendicularly or radially to the limbus (Fig. 4.4).

Iris Repositioning

The iris usually spontaneously retracts after completion of the iridectomy. If this does not occur, light pressure applied to the peripheral cornea overlying the iridectomy with a spatula or the heel of an angled cannula directed toward the pupil will facilitate repositioning

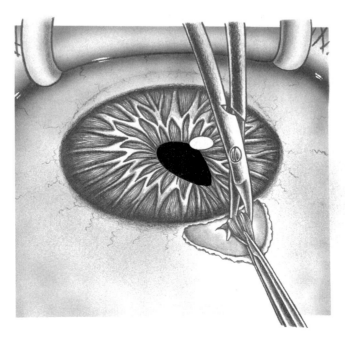
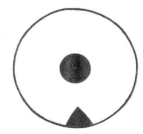

FIGURE 4.4. Peripheral iridectomy. A scissors held perpendicular to the limbus produces a narrower iridectomy with pointed contour (*inset*).

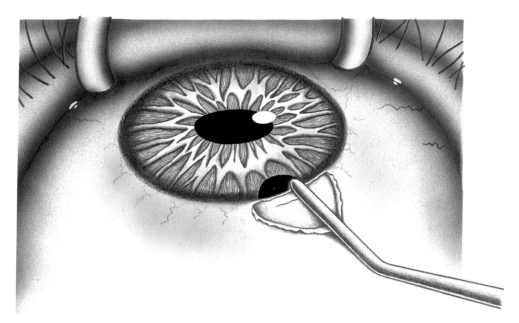

FIGURE 4.5. Peripheral iridectomy. A spatula is used to stroke the peripheral cornea and reposition the iris.

(Fig. 4.5). Alternatively, acetylcholine chloride (Miochol-E, Ciba Vision, Duluth, GA), a direct-acting miotic, injected into the anterior chamber will constrict the pupil.

Wound Closure

The limbal or clear corneal incision should be closed with one or two interrupted 10-0 nylon sutures and the knots should be buried. The conjunctiva is closed with either 10-0 nylon or 8-0 or 10-0 Vicryl (Ethicon Products Worldwide, Johnson & Johnson, Somerville, NJ) interrupted sutures (Fig. 4.6).

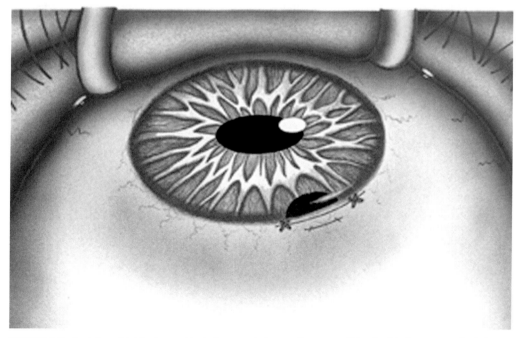

FIGURE 4.6. Peripheral iridectomy. Limbal wound closure is accomplished with interrupted 10-0 nylon sutures.

Postoperative Medications

A combination antibiotic and corticosteroid ointment is usually applied, although some surgeons prefer subconjunctival injections. A short-acting cycloplegic agent, such as cyclopentolate hydrochloride USP 1%, or ophthalmic solution should be instilled to minimize posterior synechiae formation. A patch and shield should be placed for the first day after surgery.

SURGICAL PEARLS

- Perform surgical peripheral iridectomy when corneal edema, anterior chamber inflammation, or an extremely narrow angle prevents clear visualization of the iris surface. If you cannot clearly see the iris, an iridectomy will be difficult to accomplish. Closure of an LPI associated with chronic anterior chamber inflammation is an uncommon indication for surgical peripheral iridectomy.
- Consider a limbal incision instead of a clear corneal incision. The limbal incision should extend into the anterior chamber anterior to Schwalbe's line. Posteriorly located limbal incisions may damage the iris root or ciliary body.
- Enter the anterior chamber slowly to avoid sudden decompression. If a very high intraocular pressure cannot be lowered preoperatively with medical therapy, a separate temporal paracentesis tract may be used to slowly decompress the eye.
- Avoid perforating the iris with the blade when entering the anterior chamber.
- Apply light pressure to the posterior (scleral) lip of the limbal incision to facilitate iris prolapse.
- Avoid introducing toothed forceps into the anterior chamber to grasp the iris; it may damage the cornea or lens.
- Stroke the peripheral cornea lightly in a radial direction to reposition the iris.
- Perform a smaller peripheral iridectomy rather than a larger central one. The superior border of the pupil should be deformed minimally when retracting the iris.
- Confirm that full-thickness iris tissue has been removed. Check the iridectomy specimen for the posterior pigment epithelium layer. Look for a red reflex through the iridectomy.
- Always perform an inferior peripheral iridectomy in an aphakic eye filled with silicone oil after vitrectomy. Low molecular weight silicone oil floats superiorly on the aqueous humor and may block a superiorly located iridectomy. A prophylactic inferior iridectomy should be performed in all aphakic eyes that receive silicone oil (2).
- Instill cycloplegic agents after surgery to control inflammation and to minimize posterior synechiae formation.

REFERENCES

1. Chandler PA. Peripheral iridectomy. *Arch Ophthalmol* 1964; 72:804–807.
2. Ando F. Intraocular hypertension resulting from pupillary block by silicone oil. *Am J Ophthalmol* 1985;99:87–88.

5

STANDARD TRABECULECTOMY

Trabeculectomy, the most commonly performed glaucoma filtering procedure, increases aqueous outflow through a surgical fistula into the subconjunctival space (1). To minimize complications and enhance surgical success, attention should be paid to each step of the procedure. We suggest reviewing Chapters 1 and 2 to understand the indications, rationale, and anatomy of the procedure.

CLEAR CORNEA TRACTION SUTURE

To visualize the 12:00 limbal meridian, which is the preferred surgical site, the eye must be directed inferiorly. When using topical anesthesia, the surgeon asks the patient to look downward and repeats this request throughout the procedure. We usually prefer to place a clear cornea traction suture to maintain infraduction. After rotating the eye inferiorly with two moistened cotton-tipped applicators or the heel of a muscle hook, the surgeon passes a 5-0 or 7-0 braided polyglactin 910 suture (Vicryl, J546, Ethicon Products Worldwide, Johnson & Johnson, Somerville, NJ) on a spatula needle (TG-140-8, Ethicon Products Worldwide, Johnson & Johnson, Somerville, NJ) through the peripheral corneal stroma at 50% depth (Fig. 5.1). If surgery is planned in the superior nasal or superior temporal quadrant, the suture is placed directly anterior to the scleral flap. The intracorneal suture tract should be approximately the same length as the chord width of the needle, 2 to 3 mm (Fig. 5.2).

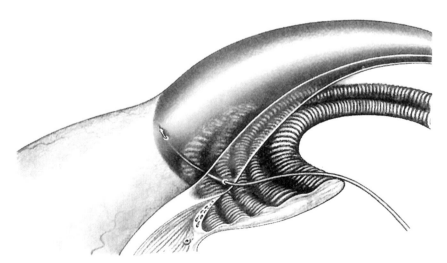

FIGURE 5.1. Clear corneal traction suture placed at 50% to 75% stromal depth.

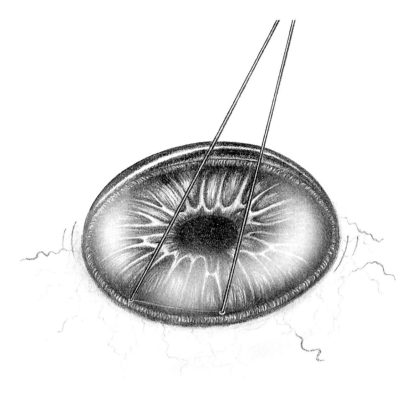

FIGURE 5.2. Superior clear corneal traction suture (11:30 to 1:00) for infra-duction.

CONJUNCTIVAL INCISION

In standard trabeculectomy, the surgeon dissects either a limbus- or a fornix-based conjunctival flap to expose the corneoscleral junction. Since neither incision provides superior intraocular pressure (IOP) control, surgeon preference guides the selection (2). Fornix-based flaps are easier to develop and usually provide better exposure than limbus-based flaps. Watertight wound closure may be more difficult to achieve with fornix-based flaps, particularly with the use of 5-fluorouracil (5-FU) and mitomycin C (MMC). The risk of intraoperative conjunctival buttonhole formation is higher with limbus-based flaps and the procedure is more time consuming.

Limbus-Based Flap

The surgeon grasps the conjunctiva near the 12:00 meridian, approximately 8 mm posterior to the limbus with a nontoothed forceps (Dressing Forceps, Product Number

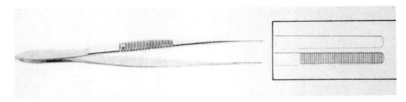

FIGURE 5.3. Serrated dressing forceps (Product Number E1400, Storz Instruments, Bausch & Lomb, Rochester, NY).

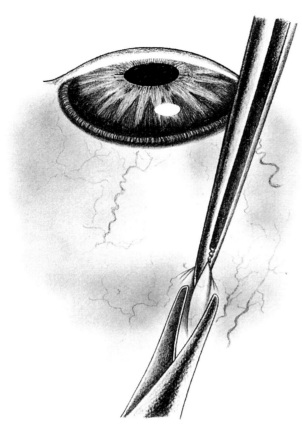

FIGURE 5.4. Limbus-based conjunctival flap with nontoothed forceps and blunt-tipped Westcott scissors (Storz Instruments, Bausch & Lomb, Rochester, NY).

E1400, Storz Instruments, Bausch & Lomb, Rochester, NY) (Fig. 5.3) to form a radial or vertical fold (Fig. 5.4). With the blades of a rounded-tip Westcott scissors (Product Number E3322, Storz Instruments, Bausch & Lomb, Rochester, NY) held perpendicular to the fold, a 2- to 3-mm circumferential cut is made through the conjunctiva without cutting Tenon's capsule or injuring the underlying superior rectus muscle (Fig. 5.4). Through this opening, the posterior tip of the scissors blade is advanced approximately 4 to 5 mm in each direction to make an 8-mm conjunctival incision (Fig. 5.5). The surgeon then grasps Tenon's capsule and cuts it with the same scissors to produce an incision approximately 2 mm anterior and parallel to the conjunctival opening (Fig. 5.6). After identifying the episclera, subconjunctival tissue is bluntly dissected anteriorly to the limbal conjunctival insertion. Episcleral adhesions to Tenon's capsule are gently cut with a sharp blade (Fig. 5.7) or bluntly teased apart with a cellulose sponge or a cotton-tipped applicator. To avoid inadvertent conjunctival perforation, particularly in eyes with extensive scarring, the conjunctival flap should be held with serrated tissue forceps and lifted perpendicularly to the episcleral surface. Adhesions between Tenon's capsule and episclera encountered approximately 2 mm posterior to the conjunctival insertion may be gently cut by stroking with a straight rounded-tip blade (Alcon Surgical Blade No. 64, Alcon Laboratories, Fort Worth, TX) (Figs. 5.8, 5.9, and 5.10). Cellulose sponges that minimize conjunctival injury should be used to retract the flap anteriorly for limbal exposure.

(*text continues on page 29*)

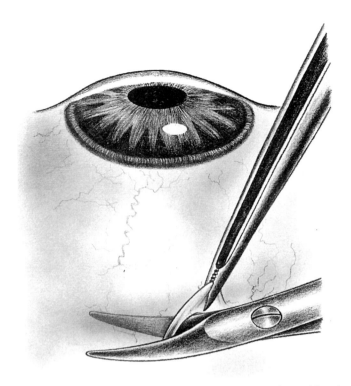

FIGURE 5.5. Limbus-based conjunctival flap extension with scissors held parallel to the conjunctival insertion, approximately 8 mm posterior to the corneoscleral junction.

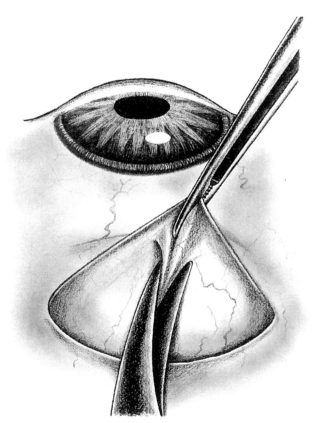

FIGURE 5.6. Tenon's capsule incision with Westcott scissors (Storz Instruments, Bausch & Lomb, Rochester, NY). Note position of the scissors held perpendicular to Tenon's capsule that has been stretched or put on tension.

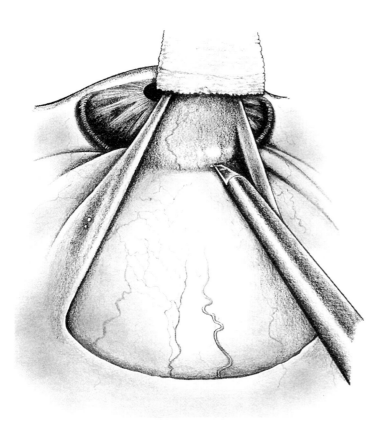

FIGURE 5.7. Disinsertion of Tenon's capsule with sharp blade. Note retraction of conjunctival flap with cellulose sponge.

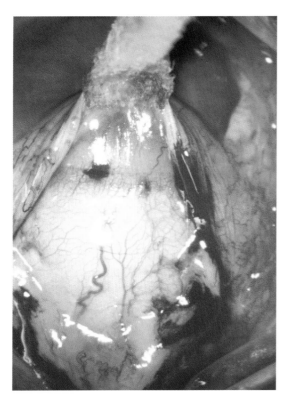

FIGURE 5.8. Limbus-based conjunctival flap before disinsertion of Tenon's capsule.

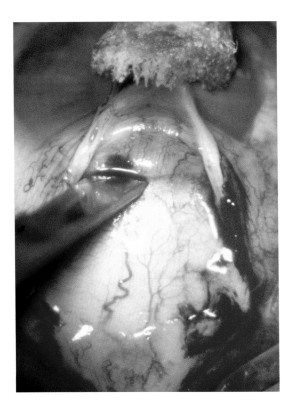

FIGURE 5.9. Disinsertion of Tenon's capsule with round blade.

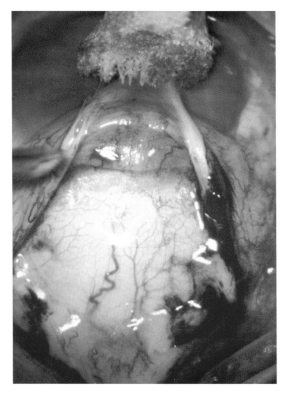

FIGURE 5.10. Appearance of limbus after disinsertion of Tenon's capsule.

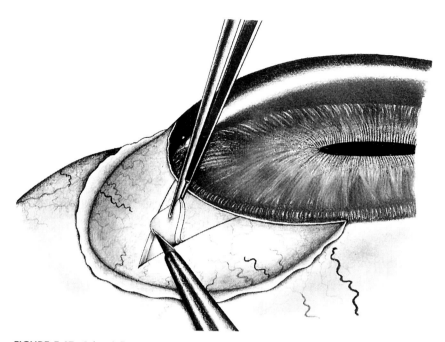

FIGURE 5.17. Scleral flap dissection. Retraction of flap toward the limbus to facilitate dissection by placing scleral fibers on stretch.

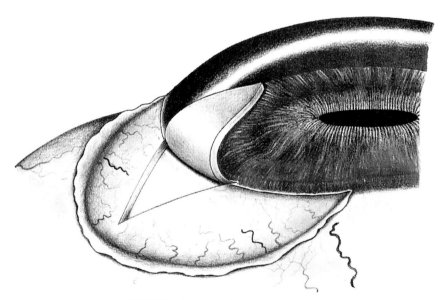

FIGURE 5.18. Completed scleral flap.

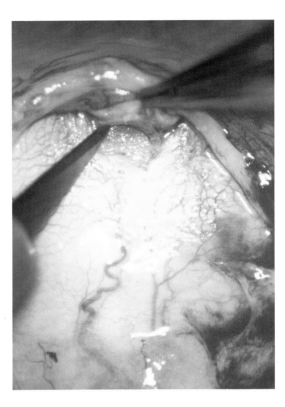

FIGURE 5.19. Scleral flap dissection into clear cornea. Note position of sharp blade facing the surgeon.

PARACENTESIS

A self-sealing paracentesis tract should be made through the temporal clear cornea before entering the anterior chamber (Fig. 5.20). Through this site, the surgeon can reform the anterior chamber and test for conjunctival wound leaks. The surgeon passes a 15-degree sharp blade through the corneal periphery to produce a beveled incision, parallel to the iris plane. Pressure applied to the globe near the limbus opposite the entry site with two

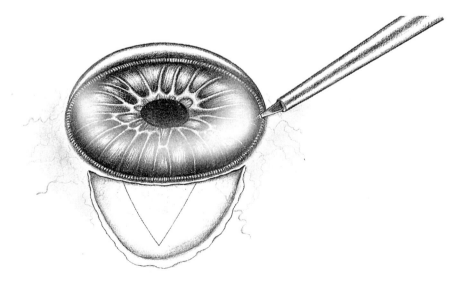

FIGURE 5.20. Paracentesis in temporal clear cornea with a sharp blade.

moistened cotton-tipped applicators stabilizes the eye. Alternatively, the paracentesis can be made with a 27-gauge needle, although this is somewhat more difficult to locate later in the procedure.

REMOVAL OF THE INNER BLOCK: SCLERECTOMY

Inner Block Removal with a Descemet's Punch

The surgeon first makes an incision to 90% corneal depth with a sharp blade held parallel to the optical axis at the anterior base of the scleral flap. The incision should be as wide as the base of the scleral flap to facilitate the punch insertion. The incision is gradually deepened with multiple shallow cuts until aqueous humor is seen (Figs. 5.21 and 5.22). Sudden decompression may cause excessive aqueous outflow and a flat or shallow anterior chamber that will complicate inner block removal. With the scleral flap elevated, the surgeon introduces a Kelly Descemet's membrane punch (Product Number E2798, Storz Instruments, Bausch & Lomb, Rochester, NY) into the middle of the incision by placing the cutting edge facing posteriorly. (Fig. 5.23). Closing the punch removes a 0.75-mm hemicircular block of limbal tissue (Figs. 5.24 and 5.25). Two or three punches are made to produce an opening approximately 2 × 1 mm. The surgeon should not exert excessive posterior force on the scleral spur; doing so could result in injury to the ciliary body and major circle of the iris. Ideally, only deep peripheral corneal stroma and Descemet's membrane anterior to the scleral spur should be removed.

Inner Block Removal with Scissors

The initial incision and anterior chamber entry are identical to the technique used with the Descemet's punch. The surgeon then makes two radial 1 mm incisions directed posteriorly at each end of the incision with straight or angled Vannas scissors (Vannas Straight

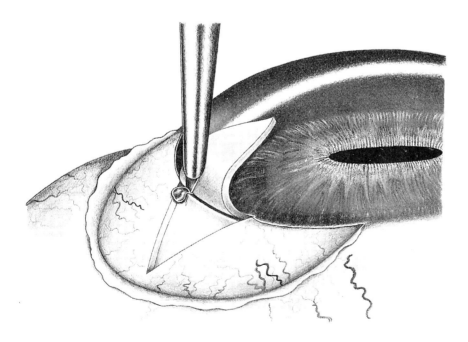

FIGURE 5.21. Inner block removal. Anterior chamber entry through peripheral clear cornea with sharp blade. Note position of blade parallel to the optical axis.

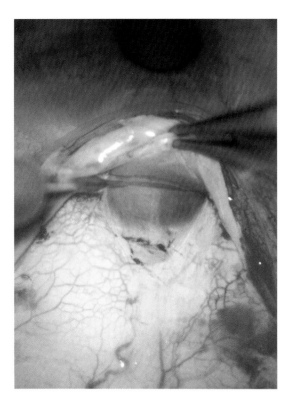

FIGURE 5.22. Inner block removal. Note blade position at anterior chamber entry through peripheral clear cornea.

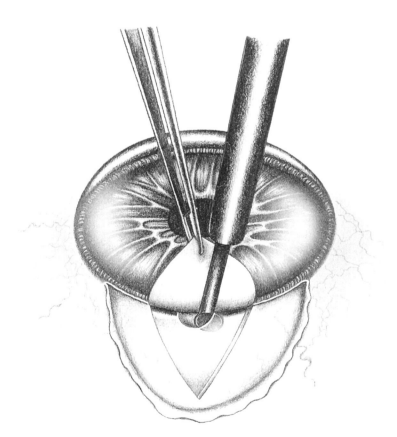

FIGURE 5.23. Inner block removal. Kelly Descemet's punch (Storz Instruments, Bausch & Lomb, Rochester, NY) produces a fistula by removing two or three bites of scleral bed anterior to scleral spur. Note position of punch held parallel to the optical axis.

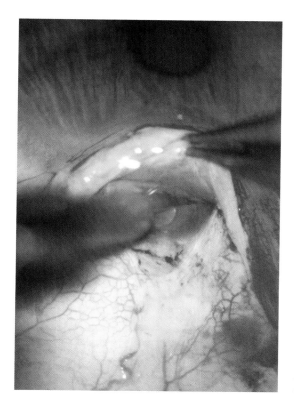

FIGURE 5.24. Inner block removal with Kelly Descemet's punch.

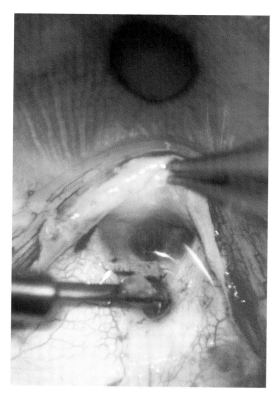

FIGURE 5.25. Completion of inner block removal.

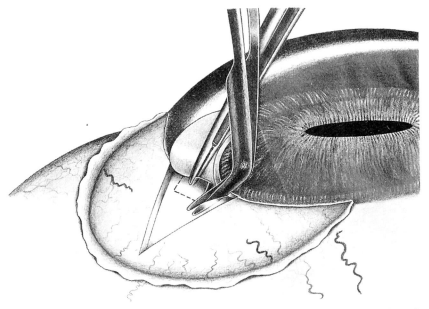

FIGURE 5.26. Inner block removal with Vannas scissors (Storz Instruments, Bausch & Lomb, Rochester, NY). Two cuts made with angled Vannas scissors perpendicular to the limbus outline the lateral margins of the inner block.

Capsulotomy Scissors, Product Number E3386 or Vannas Angled Capsulotomy Scissors Product Number E3389, Storz Instruments, Bausch & Lomb, Rochester, NY) (Fig. 5.26). The incisions should not extend beyond the scleral spur as the ciliary body and major circle of the iris may be injured. The surgeon completes the inner block excision by cutting the posterior attachment near the limbus with a Vannas scissors. The scissors are held parallel and anterior to the scleral spur and iris root (Fig. 5.27).

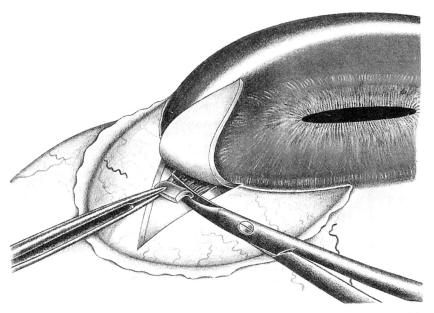

FIGURE 5.27. Inner block removal. Final cut anterior to the scleral spur with straight Vannas scissors (Storz Instruments, Bausch & Lomb, Rochester, NY) completes inner block resection.

PERIPHERAL IRIDECTOMY

After inner block removal, the peripheral iris usually spontaneously bulges or protrudes into the filtering site. The surgeon positions the opened Barraquer iris scissors (Product Number E3366, Storz Instruments, Bausch & Lomb, Rochester, NY) or Vannas scissors parallel to the limbus, grasps the iris with a 0.12-mm toothed forceps slightly anterior to the center of the inner block, and retracts it posteriorly over the posterior blade of the iris scissors (Fig. 5.28). The open scissors, held tangent to the limbus, are closed to complete the iridectomy (Figs. 5.29, 5.30, and 5.31). Ideally the surgeon does not grasp the iris with a toothed forceps within the eye and risk possible injury to the anterior lens capsule.

If the surgeon encounters excessive iris prolapse, then the lid speculum should be inspected and adjusted, if necessary, to lessen any external pressure on the globe. The firmness of the eye should be determined by applying light corneal pressure with a collagen sponge to exclude the possibility of an early intraoperative suprachoroidal hemorrhage or effusion. If no external speculum pressure is noted and the eye is soft, then a small peripheral iridotomy usually permits iris repositioning and outflow of aqueous humor from the posterior chamber. With the iris in the normal position, the peripheral iridectomy can be then safely performed. If iridotomy does not permit repositioning of the iris, gentle pressure over the peripheral cornea and scleral flap applied with a cotton-tipped applicator usually resolves the problem. Injection of a short-acting miotic, such as acetylcholine chloride intraocular solution (Miochol-E 1:100 with electrolyte diluent, OMJ Pharmaceuticals, San German, Puerto Rico), usually pulls the peripheral iris anteriorly from the filtering site.

SCLERAL FLAP CLOSURE

Three interrupted 10-0 nylon sutures close the triangular flap. The apex suture aligns the flap to the original position and should not be tied too tightly (Fig. 5.32). The two side sutures, placed near the anterior limbal base of the triangular flap, serve to direct aqueous

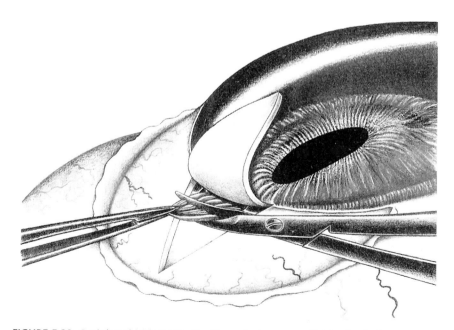

FIGURE 5.28. Peripheral iridectomy. Position of scissors parallel to the limbus.

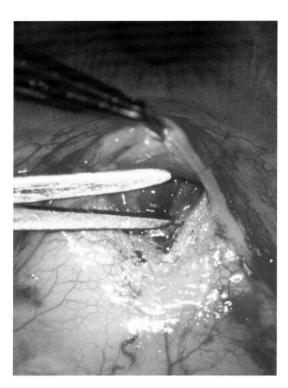

FIGURE 5.29. Peripheral iridectomy. de Wecker's scissors (Storz Instruments, Bausch & Lomb, Rochester, NY) with opened blades anterior and posterior to iridectomy site. Note position of scissors held parallel to the limbus.

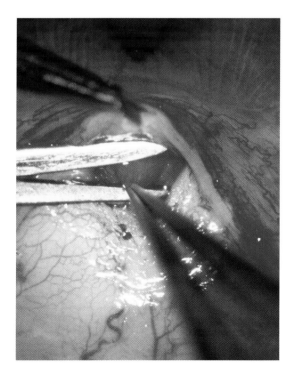

FIGURE 5.30. Peripheral iridectomy. Retraction of iris over posterior scissors blade.

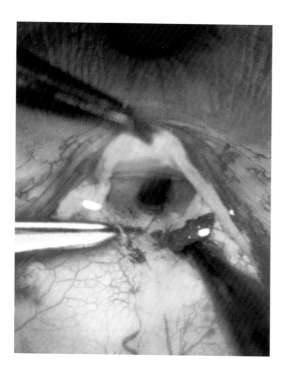

FIGURE 5.31. Peripheral iridectomy. Completion of iridectomy. Note that iridectomy width is comparable to width of the inner block.

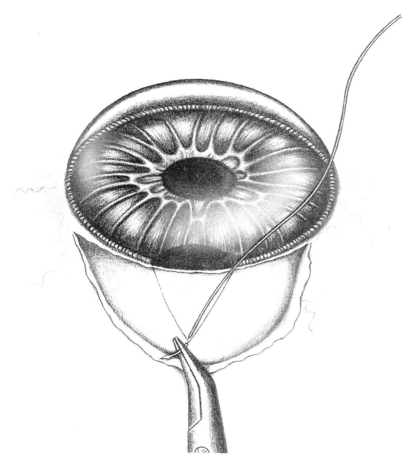

FIGURE 5.32. Scleral flap closure. Initial single interrupted 10-0 nylon suture placed at the flap apex.

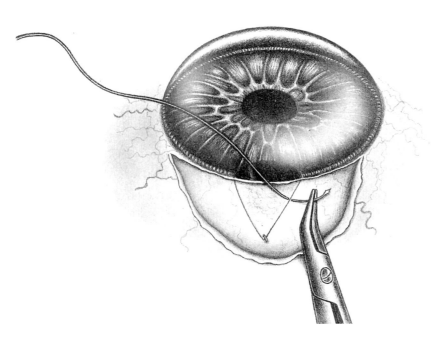

FIGURE 5.33. Scleral flap closure. Additional interrupted 10-0 nylon sutures on sides of the flap.

humor flow posteriorly (Fig. 5.33). To prevent the suture ends from perforating the overlying conjunctiva, all knots should be buried under the scleral surface with a nontoothed (e.g., Kelman-McPherson) tying forceps. The surgeon buries the knots by rotating the sutures anteriorly toward the scleral flap. The rate of aqueous humor outflow is evaluated by wiping the edge of the scleral flap with a cellulose sponge while injecting balanced salt solution through the paracentesis tract (Fig. 5.34). Suture tension should be adjusted to achieve visible aqueous outflow, normal anterior chamber depth, and IOP between 10 and 15 mm Hg.

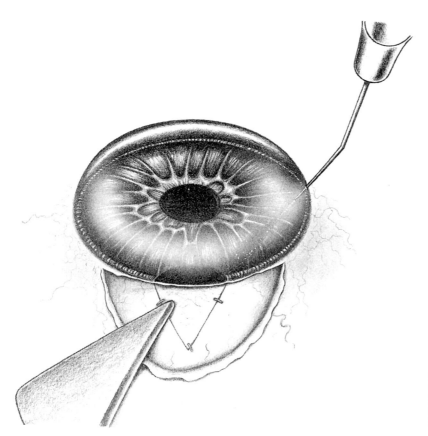

FIGURE 5.34. Assessment of aqueous humor flow. Surgeon assesses the rate of aqueous humor runoff by wiping the scleral incision with a cellulose sponge as balanced salt solution is injected through the paracentesis tract.

Square or rectangular flap closure usually requires additional sutures, depending on the size and position of the inner block, to achieve the desired aqueous runoff.

CONJUNCTIVAL CLOSURE

Limbus-Based Flap

A single continuous running 10-0 nylon Vicryl suture on a tapered-point needle (BV130-4, Ethicon Products Worldwide, Johnson & Johnson, Somerville, NJ) closes the conjunctiva and Tenon's capsule wound in a watertight fashion (Figs. 5.35 and 5.36). The surgeon may suture conjunctiva and Tenon's capsule either separately (two layer) or as one tissue (single layer) (Fig. 5.37). Two-layer closure, although more time consuming, may result in fewer wound leaks, particularly in eyes with previous conjunctival surgery (3).

Fornix-Based Flap

Interrupted 10-0 nylon horizontal mattress sutures are used to close fornix-based conjunctival flaps. Although some surgeons use absorbable sutures, we prefer 10-0 nylon because wound healing may be altered by postoperative injections of 5-FU. First, the surgeon passes the needle in a forehand manner into the anterior edge of Tenon's capsule and exits through the overlying conjunctiva. Second, he directs the needle in a backhand pass through conjunctiva and Tenon's capsule at the distal edge of the incision to enter the limbus to exit through the peripheral cornea. Finally, he passes the needle from the peripheral cornea into the limbus near the original suture site (Fig. 5.38). When the suture is tied, the knot lies buried under the conjunctiva. With excessive conjunctival retraction and scarring, the assistant may pull Tenon's capsule anteriorly with a nontoothed tissue forceps to assure proper wound apposition. The wound is reinforced with additional horizontal mattress sutures to achieve watertight closure. To check for wound leaks and buttonholes, the surgeon wipes the conjunctival incision site with a collagen sponge while injecting balanced salt solution into the anterior chamber through the paracentesis tract (Fig. 5.39). Alternatively, a contin-

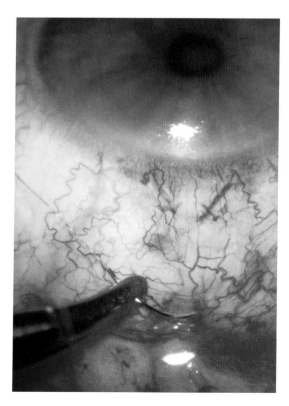

FIGURE 5.35. Single-layer closure of limbus-based flap. A running baseball-type suture closes both Tenon's capsule and conjunctival wounds.

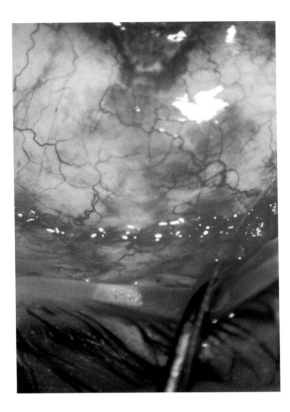

FIGURE 5.36. Single-layer closure of limbus-based flap. Completion of running suture.

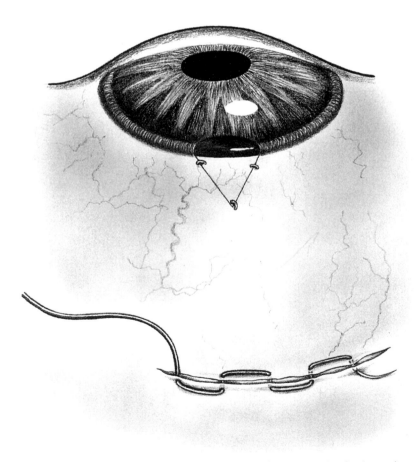

FIGURE 5.37. Single-layer closure of limbus-based flap. A running horizontal mattress suture (Greek key pattern) closes both conjunctival and Tenon's flap.

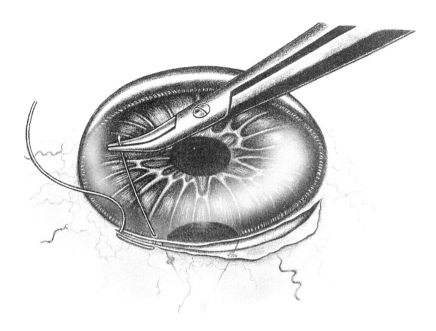

FIGURE 5.38. Single-layer closure of fornix-based flap. Interrupted horizontal mattress sutures close Tenon's capsule and conjunctiva.

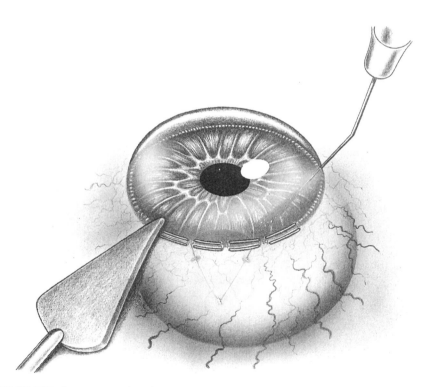

FIGURE 5.39. Assessment of conjunctival closure. Surgeon checks for watertight closure with a cellulose sponge as balanced salt solution is injected through the paracentesis tract.

uous running suture or multiple figure-of-8 sutures may be used to close the fornix-based flap. All knots should be buried to minimize patient discomfort.

END OF THE PROCEDURE

An elevated filtering bleb should be seen at the end of the procedure. Topical 1% atropine sulfate is instilled to minimize patient discomfort and to deepen the anterior chamber by providing cycloplegia. A broad-spectrum antibiotic, such as gentamicin sulfate (20 mg), and the corticosteroid dexamethasone sodium phosphate (2 mg), are usually injected sub-conjunctivally, although many surgeons do not use any postoperative antibiotic.

SURGICAL PEARLS

- Consider early trabeculectomy if medical treatment or laser surgery does not reduce IOP substantially below levels that caused optic nerve damage and visual field loss.
- Carefully determine the preoperative refraction to anticipate uncommon intraoperative and postoperative problems. Hypotony maculopathy occurs more frequently in highly myopic eyes with low scleral rigidity, particularly when 5-FU and MMC are used. Consider the use of multiple interrupted scleral flap sutures to minimize postoperative hypotony. Highly hyperopic eyes are at high risk for postoperative choroidal effusions and flat anterior chambers, particularly when nanophthalmos (dwarf eye) is present. Preoperatively perform A-scan echography to determine axial length and B-scan echography to evaluate for chorioretinal thickening. In nanophthalmic eyes, perform prophylactic inferotemporal and inferonasal sclerotomies before dissecting the scleral flap (see Chapter 8). Suture the flap more tightly than usual to minimize the likelihood of postoperative hypotony and exudative choroidal and retinal detachment.
- Place the traction suture in the clear cornea instead of under the superior rectus muscle. Take care that the needle tip does not damage conjunctival blood vessels.
- Consider the risk of postoperative wound leaks with limbus-based versus fornix-based conjunctival flaps in your experience. Limbus-based flaps require more conjunctival handling and increase the possibility of buttonhole formation. Fornix-based flaps provide a better surgical exposure and are easier to dissect, but demand meticulous wound closure. The risk of postoperative wound leaks may be greater with fornix-based flaps and 5-FU or MMC use.
- Improve exposure with limbus-based flaps by making circumferential radial relaxing incisions through Tenon's capsule near the insertion.
- Limit use of cautery to minimize thermal related tissue necrosis that might cause inflammation and stimulate wound healing.
- Remember the limbal surgical anatomy when dissecting the scleral flap. From viewpoint of the surgeon operating at the 12:00 meridian, the first uniform white zone encountered, the *sclera*, is followed by a blue–gray line, the *sclerolimbal union*. Anterior to the sclerolimbal union, a white band with fibers running parallel to the limbus marks the position of the *scleral spur*. A blue–gray zone located anterior to the scleral spur corresponds to the underlying *trabecular meshwork* that terminates in *Schwalbe's line*. Anterior to Schwalbe's line, the tissue becomes more transparent as the *peripheral corneal stroma*.
- Enter the anterior chamber through clear cornea when making the anterior incision for the inner block removal. If scissors are used to remove the block, do not cut posteriorly to the scleral spur.

- Consider making the paracentesis tract immediately after dissecting the scleral flap but before removing the inner block. A scleral flap is more easily dissected when the IOP is normal or slightly elevated. Place the paracentesis in the temporal inferior cornea, where it can be easily accessed for anterior chamber reformation if necessary.

- Do not use viscoelastic materials routinely as they interfere with the judging of aqueous humor outflow. Only consider injecting viscoelastic material in eyes with shallow anterior chambers to prevent iris prolapse after inner block removal. Remove any remaining viscoelastic before suturing the scleral flap to minimize the likelihood of a postoperative IOP spike.

- Confirm iridectomy patency by examining the specimen removed for pigment epithelium and visualizing the anterior lens capsule.

- Apply a dilute solution of fluorescein sodium to the conjunctival incision or paint the wound with fluorescein sodium strips, USP (Flourets, Chauvin Pharmaceuticals Ltd, Harold Hill, Rumford, Essex, England) and examine with a cobalt blue filter light to check for leaks, if the watertight nature of the wound is in doubt.

- Consider a combination antibiotic and corticosteroid ointment instead of a subconjunctival injection that may produce subconjunctival bleeding.

REFERENCES

1. Cairns JE. Trabeculectomy; preliminary report of a new method. *Am J Ophthalmol* 1968;66:673–679.
2. Traverso CE, Tomey KF, Antonios S. Limbal- versus fornix-based conjunctival trabeculectomy flaps. *Am J Ophthalmol* 1987;104:28–32.
3. Parrish RK II, Schiffman JC, Feuer WJ, et al. Prognosis and risk factors for early postoperative wound leaks after trabeculectomy with and without 5-fluorouracil. The Fluorouracil Filtering Surgery Study Group. *Am J Ophthalmol* 2001;132:633–640.

6

SMALL-INCISION TRABECULECTOMY

Trabeculectomy, the most popular glaucoma filtering procedure, lowers intraocular pressure (IOP) by increasing aqueous humor outflow through a surgical fistula into a conjunctival bleb. Subconjunctival and episcleral fibrosis, particularly involving Tenon's capsule, are the most common causes of long-term surgical failure. Minimizing surgical trauma may lessen postoperative scarring and improve the likelihood of bleb function. Phillips (1) and later Cairns (2) described trabeculectomy performed through a clear corneal incision to minimize conjunctival and Tenon's capsule injury. Van Buskirk suggested an additional modification to provide easier access into the subconjunctival space (3). In this chapter, we will describe a modification to Van Buskirk's technique whereby trabeculectomy is performed through a small limbal incision without dissecting a peripheral corneal flap (4). A recent report compares conventional trabeculectomy and the small incision trabeculectomy that avoids Tenon's capsule (5).

ANATOMY

Tenon's capsule inserts into the scleral surface 1.5 to 2.0 mm posterior to the limbus. By approaching the sclera through a small conjunctival peritomy, this 1.5- to 2.0-mm potential space, may be entered without cutting through the capsule. By avoiding dissection and cauterization of Tenon's capsule and episclera, stimuli to wound healing are reduced.

SURGICAL TECHNIQUE

Anesthesia

Although either topical or peribulbar anesthesia may be used, the topical anesthesia is preferred. With peribulbar anesthesia, a 5-0 or 7-0 polyglactin 910 suture (Vicryl, J546, Ethicon Products Worldwide, Johnson & Johnson, Somerville, NJ) on a side-cutting spatula needle (TG-140-8) in the peripheral corneal stroma near the 12:00 meridian is used to rotate the globe inferiorly and to expose the superior limbus. If topical anesthesia is used, 0.5% proparacaine hydrochloride or 4% lidocaine drops are instilled and the patient is asked to look down.

Initial Limbal Incision

A 2.0-mm peritomy is made at the conjunctival insertion without cutting Tenon's capsule (Fig 6.1). In the space between the insertion of the conjunctiva and the attachment of Tenon's capsule, a 2.0-mm linear incision, approximately one-third to one-half limbal thickness, is made near the conjunctival incision (Fig 6.2).

Intrascleral Pocket

A 1.75-mm-wide spatula blade (BD EdgeAhead crescent knife, 1.75 mm, angled 60 degrees bevel up, Product Number 581137, Becton–Dickinson Ophthalmic Systems, Franklin Lakes, NJ) is used to develop an intrascleral pocket posteriorly (Fig 6.3). The

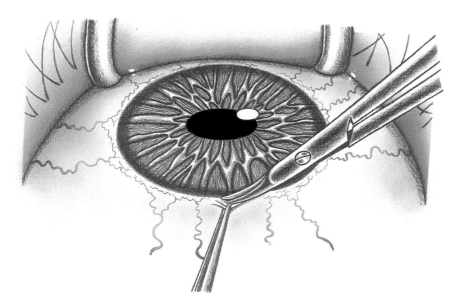

FIGURE 6.1. A 2.0-mm fornix-based conjunctival flap without Tenon's capsule incision.

width of spatula blade chosen may be conveniently varied to alter the width of the peritomy, limbal incision, and scleral pocket, such as with a 1.0-mm blade (Huco Vision SA, St. Blaise, Switzerland).

Connecting the Intrascleral Pocket to the Sub-Tenon's Space

The tip of a 27-gauge needle is bent over the lumen to produce a pointed cutting edge, similar to a cystotome. The bent needle on a tuberculin syringe filled with balanced salt solution (BSS, Alcon Laboratories, Fort Worth, TX) is passed into the intrascleral pocket with the tip oriented parallel to the floor of the flap. After reaching the deepest extent of the flap, the needle tip is rotated anteriorly 90 degrees, which results in cutting of the scle-

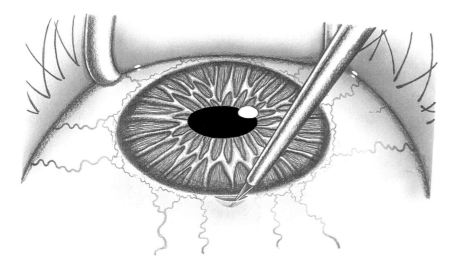

FIGURE 6.2. Anterior corneal–limbal incision at one-third to one-half depth. (From Lerner SF. Small incision trabeculectomy avoiding Tenon's capsule. A new procedure for glaucoma surgery. *Ophthalmology* 1997;104:1237–1241, with permission.)

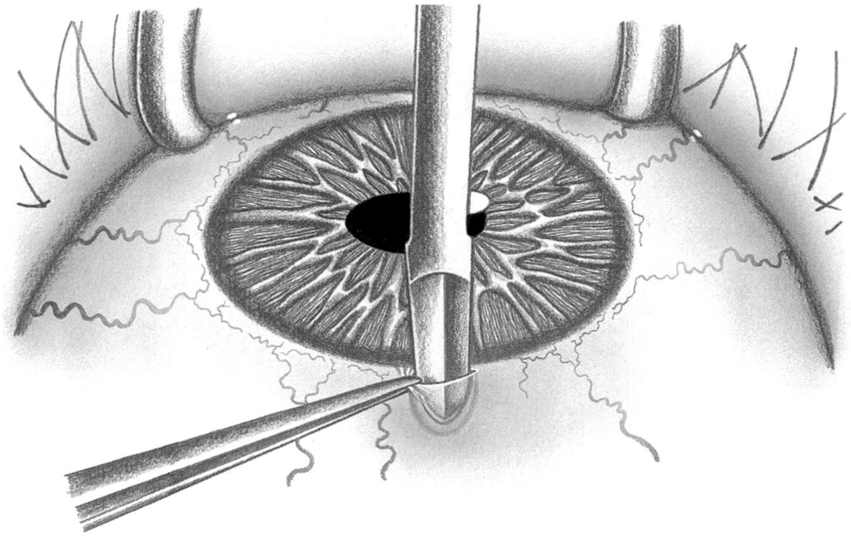

FIGURE 6.3. Scleral flap dissection with spatula blade to develop intrascleral pocket posteriorly. (From Lerner SF. Small incision trabeculectomy avoiding Tenon's capsule. A new procedure for glaucoma surgery. *Ophthalmology* 1997;104:1237–1241, with permission.)

ral pocket roof and entry into the sub-Tenon's space, posterior to its insertion (Figs. 6.4 and 6.5). The correct position of the bent needle tip may be confirmed by direct visualization and by injecting BSS, to elevate a bleb in sub-Tenon's space. The incision is enlarged by gently moving the needle tip in a side-to-side direction.

Anterior Chamber Entry

Following creation of a self-sealing clear corneal paracentesis tract, the anterior chamber is entered after the initial limbal incision has been deepened with a sharp blade (Fig. 6.6).

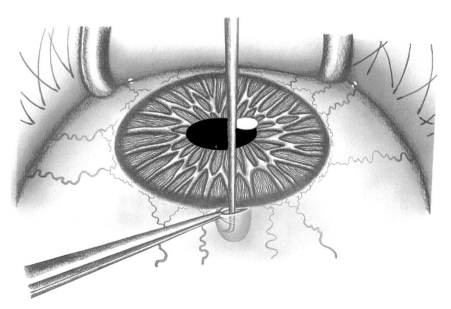

FIGURE 6.4. Cystotome position at apex of scleral pocket before incision of scleral roof. (From Lerner SF. Small incision trabeculectomy avoiding Tenon's capsule. A new procedure for glaucoma surgery. *Ophthalmology* 1997;104:1237–1241, with permission.)

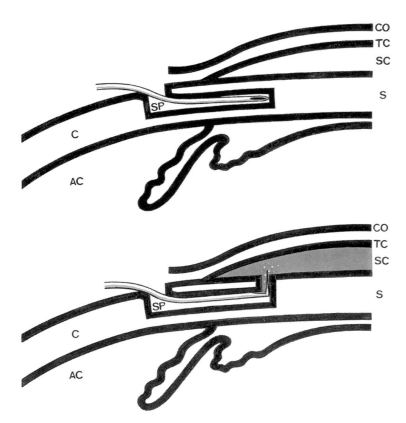

FIGURE 6.5. Diagram of cystotome inside the scleral pocket before rotation and incision of scleral pocket roof (superior figure) and after rotation of cystotome tip through the scleral pocket roof and injection of balanced salt solution into sub-Tenon's space (inferior figure). C, cornea; AC, anterior chamber; SP, scleral pocket; S, sclera; SC, sub-Tenon's space; TC, Tenon's capsule; CO, conjunctiva. (From Lerner SF. Small incision trabeculectomy avoiding Tenon's capsule. A new procedure for glaucoma surgery. *Ophthalmology* 1997;104: 1237–1241, with permission.)

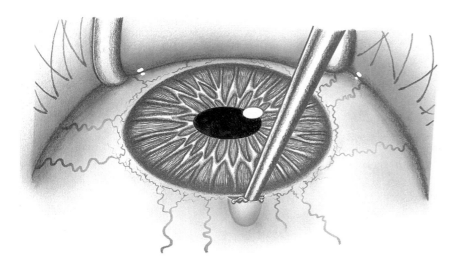

FIGURE 6.6. Deepening of initial corneal–limbal incision to enter the anterior chamber.

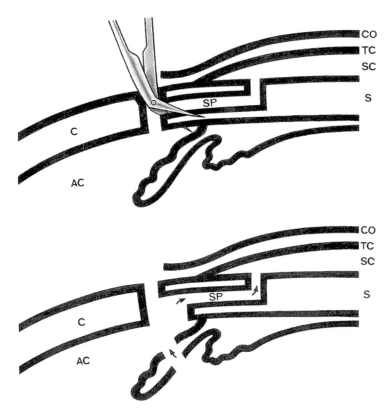

FIGURE 6.7. Resection of scleral pocket floor with Vannas scissors (Storz Instruments, Bausch & Lomb, Rochester, NY) (superior figure). Passage of aqueous humor through the fistula into sub-Tenon's space (inferior figure). C, cornea; AC, anterior chamber; SP, scleral pocket; S, sclera; SC, sub-Tenon's space; TC, Tenon's capsule; CO, conjunctiva. (From Lerner SF. Small incision trabeculectomy avoiding Tenon's capsule. A new procedure for glaucoma surgery. *Ophthalmology* 1997;104:1237–1241, with permission.)

Inner Block Removal and Peripheral Iridectomy

Angled Vannas scissors or a Kelly Descemet's membrane punch (Storz Instruments, Bausch & Lomb, Rochester, NY) are used to excise a fragment of the floor of the pocket (Figs. 6.7 and 6.8). Care should be taken to avoid cutting the scleral pocket roof. Direct visualization of the insertion of the Vannas scissors or the Descemet's punch before cutting the floor of the pocket will minimize this complication. A peripheral iridectomy is performed in the manner previously described (see Chapter 5).

Wound Closure

The corneal lip of the incision is sutured to the roof of the pocket with two bites of a running 10-0 nylon suture in a watertight manner (Fig. 6.9). The conjunctiva is closed with either running or interrupted mattress sutures of 10-0 nylon (Fig. 6.10).

Antibiotics and Corticosteroids

A broad-spectrum antibiotic and corticosteroid are usually administered, either topically or subconjunctivally, and the eye is patched. A broad diffuse bleb develops posteriorly that is not limited by scarring associated with a limbus-based flap incision (Figs. 6.11 and 6.12).

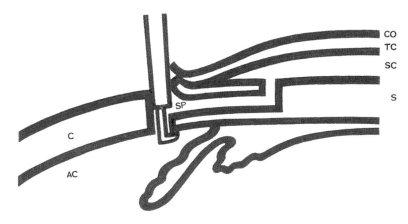

FIGURE 6.8. Resection of scleral pocket floor with a Kelly Descemet's punch (Storz Instruments, Bausch & Lomb, Rochester, NY). C, cornea; AC, anterior chamber; SP, scleral pocket; S, sclera; SC, sub-Tenon's space; TC, Tenon's capsule; CO, conjunctiva.

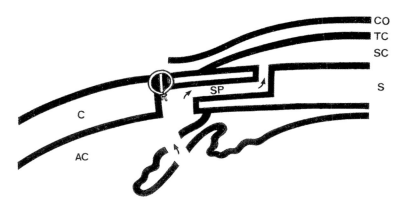

FIGURE 6.9. Anterior limbal wound with two bites of a running 10-0 nylon suture. (From Lerner SF. Small incision trabeculectomy avoiding Tenon's capsule. A new procedure for glaucoma surgery. *Ophthalmology* 1997;104: 1237–1241, with permission.)

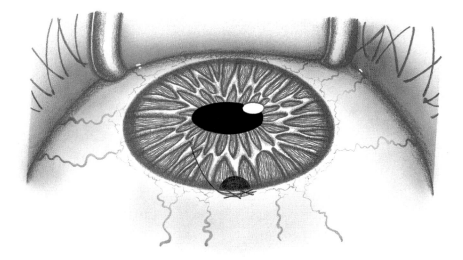

FIGURE 6.10. Conjunctiva closure with a running 10-0 nylon suture. (From Lerner SF. Small incision trabeculectomy avoiding Tenon's capsule. A new procedure for glaucoma surgery. *Ophthalmology* 1997;104:1237–1241, with permission.)

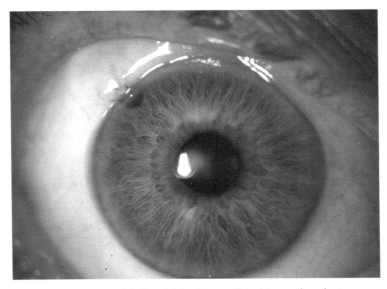

FIGURE 6.11. Broad diffuse bleb with small-incision trabeculectomy.

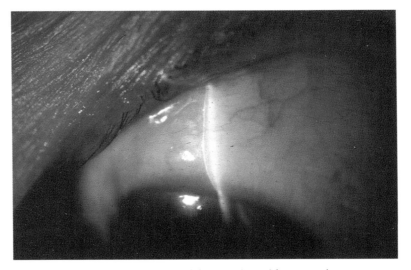

FIGURE 6.12. Posterior bleb extension without scarring.

SURGICAL PEARLS

- Anticipate low-lying diffuse blebs that are best seen with the narrow beam of the slit lamp.
- Rotate the bent 27-gauge needle anteriorly very carefully to avoid trauma to the flap and overlying conjunctiva.
- Enter the anterior chamber with the posterior blade tip of the Vannas scissors and carefully excise a fragment of the floor of the scleral pocket. If a Descemet's membrane punch is used, do not damage the roof of the pocket.
- Pass sutures superficially in the corneal incision to avoid closing the underlying fistula. This incision must be watertight to direct aqueous humor flow through the scleral pocket into the sub-Tenon's space.
- Inject 5 mg of 5-fluorouracil (0.1 mL of a standard commercial dilution, 50 mg/mL) mixed with 0.1 mL of BSS into the scleral pocket before entering the anterior chamber when treating patients with poor prognoses.
- Reduce complications of bleeding by selecting an area of sclera that does not contain perforating blood vessels. These vessels are usually associated with a ring of pigment at the site of scleral perforation (Axenfeld neurovascular loop).
- Stop bleeding associated with scleral pocket dissection or rotation of the bent 27-gauge needle by applying external pressure to the area with a cotton-tipped applicator.

REFERENCES

1. Phillips CI. Trabeculectomy "Ab externo." *Trans Ophthalmol Soc UK* 1968; 88:681–691.
2. Cairns JE. Clear-cornea trabeculectomy. *Trans Ophthalmol Soc UK* 1985;104:142–145.
3. Van Buskirk EM. Trabeculectomy without conjunctival incision. *Am J Ophthalmol* 1992;113:145–153.
4. Lerner SF. Small-incision trabeculectomy avoiding Tenon's capsule; a new procedure for glaucoma surgery. *Ophthalmology* 1997;104:1237–1241.
5. Das JC, Sharma P, Chaudhuri Z, et al. A comparative study of small incision trabeculectomy avoiding Tenon's capsule with conventional trabeculectomy. *Ophth Surg Lasers* 2002;33:30–36.

7

INTRAOPERATIVE COMPLICATIONS OF TRABECULECTOMY

Many postoperative complications, such as hypotony and shallow anterior chamber, occur as a direct result of poor surgical technique involving scleral flap dissection, inner block removal, or conjunctival closure (1). In this chapter we describe how to minimize intraoperative complications beginning with the anesthesia and proceeding through each step of the procedure.

ANESTHESIA: RETROBULBAR HEMORRHAGE

Acute retrobulbar hemorrhage presents as proptosis associated with subconjunctival hemorrhage, discoloration of the lids, and a very hard eye immediately after retrobulbar or peribulbar injection. Very high intraocular pressure (IOP), particularly in eyes with advanced glaucomatous optic neuropathy, can compromise the blood flow to the optic nerve. In these eyes, lateral canthotomy with lateral cantholysis should be performed and intravenous mannitol (0.5 to 1.0 g/kg body weight of a 10% or 20% solution at a rate of 4 mL per minute) administered. In view of the high external pressure on the globe and the risk of possible extrusion of intraocular contents, filtering surgery should be postponed and rescheduled after complete absorption of the hemorrhage. Systemic arterial hypertension, capillary fragility, and anticoagulation may predispose to this complication. The injection of peribulbar anesthetics with a blunt-tipped 18-gauge cannula through a small conjunctival incision may reduce the likelihood of injuring orbital blood vessels.

CORNEAL TRACTION SUTURE COMPLICATIONS

The globe may be rotated inferiorly without risk of injuring the conjunctiva or underlying superior rectus muscle if the surgeon uses a clear cornea traction suture. Two complications may occur as a result improper suture placement. If the suture is passed too superficially, it may pull through the anterior corneal stroma when force is applied. (Fig. 7.1). If this occurs, the suture should be removed and placed more deeply. If the suture is passed too deeply and perforates the cornea, the anterior chamber may become shallow and complicate the scleral flap dissection (Fig. 7.2). Immediately after passing the suture, the exit site through the cornea should be checked for aqueous leakage with a dry cellulose sponge. If the surgeon identifies a perforation, a paracentesis should be performed and balanced salt solution (BSS) or a viscoelastic material injected to maintain normal anterior chamber depth. We do not perform the paracentesis before cutting the flap, as dissection at the desired depth is easier when IOP is moderately elevated (i.e., 20 to 30 mm Hg). Intraoperative 5-fluorouracil (5-FU) and mitomycin C (MMC) should be administered only in eyes with poor prognoses in view of the increased risk of anterior chamber penetration with potentially toxic drugs.

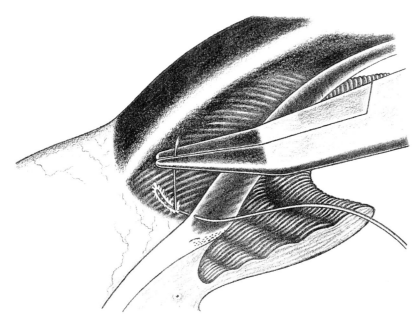

FIGURE 7.1. Superficial corneal traction suture placement. Inadvertent tearing of corneal traction suture through overlying thin corneal stroma.

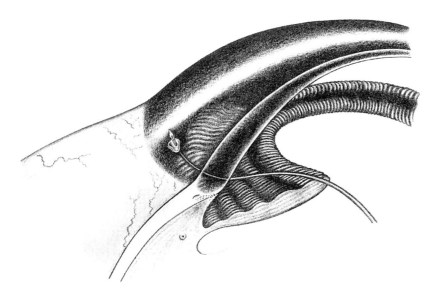

FIGURE 7.2. Excessively deep corneal traction suture. Inadvertent anterior chamber entry with very deep needle passage.

CONJUNCTIVAL COMPLICATIONS

The conjunctiva should be handled with a nontoothed forceps and dissected with blunt instruments to minimize bleeding and accidental perforation. Cautery to episclera vessels should be performed after the conjunctiva has been retracted to avoid thermal damage. Limbus-based flaps are more likely to be associated with buttonhole formation than fornix-based flaps. This risk of inadvertent perforation or buttonhole is greatest in previously operated eyes that have extensive subconjunctival scarring. To preoperatively determine the extent of fibrosis at the intended filtering site and to assess conjuntival mobility, a cotton-tipped applicator is used. To define the extent of scarring before selecting the filtering site, sterile balanced saline may be injected into the subconjunctival space through a 25-gauge needle. The location of the injection should correspond to the site of the conjunctival incision when using a limbus-based flap. The small hole produced by the 25-gauge needle tip will permit the tip of blunt Westcott scissors (Storz Instruments, Bausch & Lomb, Rochester, NY) to enter the subconjunctival space. If smaller needles are used, identification of the perforation site becomes difficult. Throughout the procedure, the conjunctiva should be inspected for tears or holes. The assistant should frequently moisten the conjunctiva with BSS to prevent drying that may predispose to buttonhole formation. At the end of the procedure, the surgeon paints the conjunctival surface and incision with either sterile dilute fluorescein sodium solution or a moistened fluorescin sodium strip, USP (Fluorets, Chauvin Pharmaceuticals Ltd., Essex, UK) to assess the adequacy of closure (Seidel test). BSS is injected through the paracentesis tract to identify leaks, reform the anterior chamber, and elevate the bleb. Any leak should be repaired before leaving the operating room. Excessive aqueous humor leakage may lead to postoperative complications of hypotony, such as cataract formation, choroidal detachment, and corneal endothelial damage. Furthermore, leaks may prevent bleb formation and lead to scarring by preventing the mechanical separation of healing subconjunctival and episcleral surfaces.

Tears and buttonholes should be closed with either 8-0 braided Vicryl (Ethicon Products Worldwide, Johnson & Johnson, Somerville, NJ) or 10-0 nylon suture on a tapered-point needle. Spatula tip needles should not be used because they cut slits that may leak around each suture. Single or multiple horizontal mattress sutures that produce minimal tension on the wound may be used (Fig. 7.3). With unusually large buttonholes, a running horizontal mattress (Greek key pattern) suture may be used. The surgeon should also test for wound leaks in the immediate postoperative period and manage them promptly to minimize such complications.

SCLERAL FLAP COMPLICATIONS

During trabeculectomy the surgeon faces the important question of how thick to make the scleral flap. Both excessively thin and thick flaps produce complications. If the flap is too thin, then it may tear partially or completely (amputated flap) (Fig. 7.4). After recognizing the tear, the surgeon may suture the flap to the anterior limbal tissue and redirect the dissection more posteriorly or simply dissect another scleral flap. Usually dissection of a new flap is preferable. Scleral flap tears are difficult to repair in a predictable manner and are often associated with excessive filtration. This is particularly true with intraoperative MMC or 5-FU use because both interfere with wound healing. If the surgeon plans to use 5-FU or MMC, then an additional autologous or glycerin-preserved scleral patch should be used to repair the flap. If preserved tissue is not available, a 50% to 70% partial thickness freehand graft should be cut from the adjacent sclera. The width of the graft should be slightly longer than the length of the tear. The graft is sewn over the tear with a horizontal mattress suture. The surgeon should place the horizontal suture bites lateral to the edge of the flap bed.

If this complication occurs in the only area suited for a trabeculectomy, the surgeon may repair the tear and continue with trabeculectomy or implant a glaucoma drainage

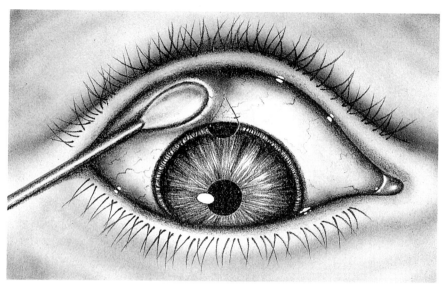

FIGURE 8.2. Postoperative wound distortion with cotton-tipped applicator. Force generated with cotton-tip application displaces the scleral bed posteriorly relative to the position of the scleral flap.

may produce thermal injury and inadvertent perforation. If conjunctival hyperemia obscures the view, apraclonidine (Iopidine, Alcon, Fort Worth, TX) may be applied to constrict the vessels. The surgeon focuses the argon laser beam (300 to 800 mW power, 0.02 to 0.2 second duration, and a 50- to 100-μm spot size) on the most peripheral point of suture entry into the sclera. If the bleb does not spontaneously elevate after one suture has been cut, light massage is performed to elevate the bleb. Suturelysis performed within the first 3 postoperative days usually lowers IOP and promotes bleb formation, if neither intraoperative mitomycin C (MMC) nor 5-FU was given. If intraoperative 5-FU has been applied, suturelysis within the first 7 postoperative days is usually successful. After intra-

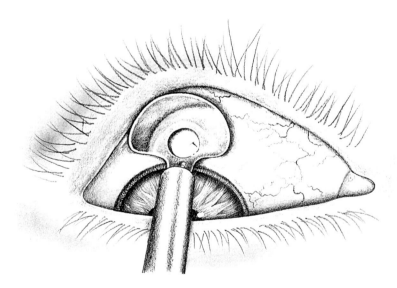

FIGURE 8.3. Suturelysis. Argon or diode laser energy is used to cut tight 10-0 nylon sutures in the scleral flap that prevent adequate aqueous humor outflow. Sutures should be cut at the most peripheral point of scleral entry relative to the limbus.

operative MMC application, suturelysis may be successful if performed as long as 6 weeks after the surgery.

Needling of the Bleb and Elevation of the Scleral Flap

If the bleb remains flat and the IOP elevated after massage and suturelysis, scarring at the episcleral surface is the most likely cause of failure. The surgeon may elevate the scleral flap with the tip of a 25-gauge needle that has been passed under the conjunctiva though the peripheral entry site. Sterile balanced salt solution (BSS) or anesthetic may be injected into the subconjunctival space to elevate the bleb and lessen the chance of perforation. To minimize further scarring, 5-FU may be injected into the subconjunctival space at a site distant from the bleb site (see Chapter 9).

ELEVATED IOP, FLAT ANTERIOR CHAMBER, AND FLAT BLEB

To determine the treatment plan a decision must be made as to whether pupillary block, annular choroidal detachment, suprachoroidal hemorrhage, or malignant glaucoma is present.

Pupillary Block

Pupillary block is associated with iris bombé configuration. The central anterior chamber depth is usually moderately shallow and the peripheral iris touches the cornea. Papillary block is treated with laser or surgical iridectomy (Chapter 4). Plateau iris syndrome, an uncommon form of angle closure that occurs in the presence of a patent peripheral iridectomy, is usually managed with peripheral iridoplasty to thermally pull the iris from the trabecular meshwork.

Postoperative Suprachoroidal Hemorrhage

Delayed postoperative suprachoroidal hemorrhage usually presents as acute and severe uniocular pain, nausea, and sudden loss of visual acuity (Fig. 8.4). Postoperative

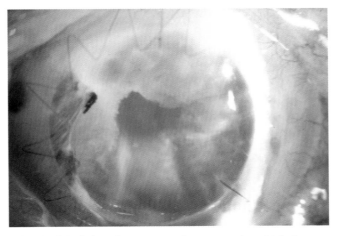

FIGURE 8.4. Delayed postoperative suprachoroidal hemorrhage. Severe ocular pain and nausea associated with sudden loss of vision in an elderly man after trabeculectomy. (Reprinted from Parrish RK II, ed. *University of Miami Bascom Palmer Eye Institute Atlas of Ophthalmology.* Philadelphia: Current Medicine, 2000:226, with permission.)

hypotony and increased preoperative IOP are risk factors for the development of this serious postoperative complication. This condition results in peripheral iridocorneal and central lenticular corneal contact (flat chamber). Blood in the suprachoroidal space, posterior to the scleral spur, rotates the ciliary body anteriorly about its point of fixation to the scleral spur. Transillumination of the eye with a muscle light (Transilluminator, Welch Allyn, Skaneateles Falls, NY) will show loss of the red reflex, and echography will demonstrate blood in the suprachoroidal space. Oral or intravenous analgesia is usually required for pain relief. Cycloplegia, topical corticosteroids, and carbonic anhydrase inhibitors are also helpful in lowering IOP and reducing discomfort. Drainage of a choroidal hemorrhage should not be attempted until clot dissolution can be demonstrated echographically, usually within 2 to 4 weeks (6). The preferred approach is pars plana vitrectomy which facilitates drainage and maintains IOP. If the hemorrhage has extended through the retina (hemorrhagic retinal detachment), the prognosis for return of vision is very poor. Limited suprachoroidal hemorrhages that do not involve the posterior pole may spontaneously absorb and do not require drainage.

Aqueous Misdirection (Malignant Glaucoma)

Postoperative diversion of aqueous humor into the vitreous cavity has been called malignant glaucoma, aqueous misdirection, ciliolenticular and vitreolenticular block glaucoma. In this condition the lens iris diaphragm is pushed anteriorly, resulting in flattening of the central anterior chamber, angle closure, sudden and high IOP elevation, and severe pain. Eyes after acute angle closure glaucoma are at a high risk to develop this complication. B-scan echography demonstrates the forward displacement of the lens-iris diaphragm without ciliary body or choroidal detachment. Medical treatment to suppress aqueous humor formation, cycloplegia, and systemic hyperosmotic agents resolves the complication in approximately 50% of eyes. If medical treatment fails, disruption of the anterior hyaloid face with Nd:YAG laser may reestablish the forward flow of aqueous humor. If this occurs in pseudophakic eyes, posterior capsulotomy must be performed as well. If medical and laser therapy do not deepen the anterior chamber, pars plana vitrectomy with disruption of the anterior hyaloid face should be performed. If pars plana vitrectomy fails to resolve the flat chamber, a repeat vitrectomy and lensectomy should be performed.

Annular Choroidal Detachment

Annular choroidal detachment may be mistaken for malignant glaucoma. In both conditions the anterior chamber is flat and the IOP is elevated without a visible bleb. High-resolution B-scan echography or ultrasonic biomicroscopy demonstrates a low-lying peripheral annular choroidal effusion posterior to the scleral spur. Treatment with cycloplegic agents, hyperosmotics, and aqueous suppressants usually resolves the condition. If medical treatment fails, drainage of the choroidal detachment may hasten absorption and anterior chamber reformation (7).

ELEVATED IOP, NORMAL ANTERIOR CHAMBER DEPTH, AND ELEVATED BLEB

Encapsulation of the filtering bleb, also known as Tenon's cyst, exteriorized anterior chamber, or cocoon bleb, is characterized by a prominently distended and vascularized conjunctival elevation without epithelial microcysts (8) (Fig. 8.5). Scarring of subconjunctival tissue around the filtering site and on the inner (subconjunctival) bleb surface prevents the passage of aqueous humor through the bleb wall. The encapsulation may involve the entire bleb cavity or only a portion of it.

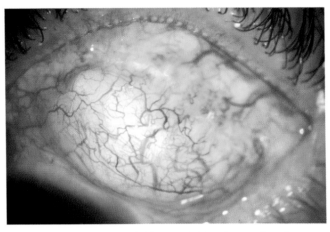

FIGURE 8.5. Encapsulated filtering bleb after trabeculectomy. Note highly elevated profile and intense vascularization. (Reprinted from Parrish RK II, ed. *University of Miami Bascom Palmer Eye Institute Atlas of Ophthalmology* Philadelphia: Current Medicine, 2000:227, with permission.)

Encapsulated blebs usually spontaneously resolve or respond to medical therapy with aqueous suppressants; however, resolution may take 2 or 3 months. Initially prominent bleb vascularization decreases after several weeks. Topical corticosteroids may be administered to reduce inflammation but probably do not hasten resolution of the encapsulated bleb. Digital massage may be used to force aqueous humor through the wall of the bleb into the surrounding subconjunctival space. Massage can be performed as described previously or by pressing a cotton-tipped applicator soaked with topical anesthetic directly over the cyst. When the technique has been successfully completed, aqueous humor flows into the subconjunctival space outside the boundaries of the cyst and the IOP is lowered. If the cyst does not respond to conservative medical therapy, either incisional (needling) or excisional surgical revision may improve functioning of the bleb.

Needling of Encapsulated Bleb

Needling is performed to lower IOP in the immediate postoperative period if the patient cannot tolerate medical therapy or if an urgent need to lower IOP exists. Although the procedure may be performed with the surgical microscope in the operating room, it is usually done at the slit lamp. After applying topical anesthesia, the surgeon introduces a 25-gauge needle on a tuberculin syringe into the subconjunctival space approximately 3 mm from the posterior border of the cyst. Approximately 0.2 to 0.3 mL of BSS or 1% lidocaine without epinephrine may be injected to separate the overlying conjunctiva from the bleb wall and minimize conjunctival perforation. Although sometimes helpful, this fluid may interfere with monitoring of bleb size after needling. The needle tip is carefully advanced to the wall of the encapsulated bleb and the bleb cavity is entered with multiple punctures under direct observation. The tip is slowly moved to produce a slit-like opening in the bleb wall (Fig. 8.6). After entering the cavity, the bleb usually spontaneously expands posteriorly along the needle tract and the anterior chamber may shallow. After the needling, subconjunctival injections of 5-FU may reduce subsequent wound healing and bleb fibrosis (see Chapter 9). If the needling is not effective in establishing a diffuse bleb, surgical revision of the encapsulated bleb may be performed (see Chapter 10).

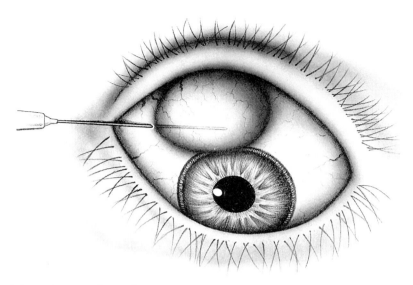

FIGURE 8.6. Needling of encapsulated bleb. A 25-gauge needle enters the conjunctiva 2 mm peripheral to the bleb wall.

LOW IOP, NORMAL OR SHALLOW ANTERIOR CHAMBER, AND FLAT BLEB

Conjunctival wound leaks and serous choroidal detachments are associated with the clinical presentation of low IOP, normal or shallow anterior chamber, and flat bleb. Hypotony, less than 10 mm Hg, without a visible bleb, should alert the surgeon to the possibility of a leak and the Seidel test should be performed. If no leak is found, following blinking and after application of light pressure to the globe through the lid, the test should be repeated. The IOP and the anterior chamber depth may be normal if leakage is minimal and the choroidal detachments are small. If leakage is detected, pressure patching with two sterile eye pads to maintain lid closure is performed. Usually 1% atropine sulfate and a combination corticosteroid/antibiotic ointment are applied, with the patch remaining in place for 24 to 48 hours. Alternatively, a large soft contact lens (Kontur Kontacts, Richmond, CA) may be used to protect the wound from the abrasive effect of upper lid movement. Occasionally light applications of a large spot size (200 μm), low-power (200 mW), long-duration (200 msec) argon or diode laser energy to the leak site may produce local thermal effects and stimulate healing. This is most likely to be successful if fine conjunctival vessels are present which will absorb the argon laser energy.

If the leak does not resolve with conservative treatment or if central corneal lenticular contact develops (flat chamber), surgical repair and anterior chamber reformation should be performed as soon as possible. Braided 8-0 Vicryl or 9-0 Vicryl (Ethicon Products Worldwide, Johnson & Johnson, Somerville, NJ) or 10-0 nylon sutures are used to close the leak as described in Chapter 7.

An inadvertently created cyclodialysis cleft is a rare cause of low IOP, normal or shallow anterior chamber, and flat bleb. Gonioscopy will demonstrate the cleft, although visualization is often difficult though corneal folds.

LOW IOP, SHALLOW OR FLAT ANTERIOR CHAMBER, AND ELEVATED BLEB

Overfiltration of aqueous humor through the filtering site is the most likely cause of low IOP, shallow or flat anterior chamber, and elevated bleb. A loosely sutured scleral flap and

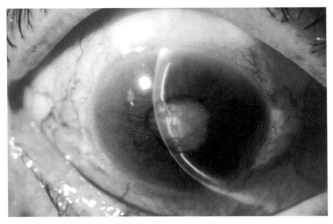

FIGURE 8.7. Flat anterior chamber after trabeculectomy with cataract formation. (Reprinted from Parrish RK II, ed. *University of Miami Bascom Palmer Eye Institute Atlas of Ophthalmology.* Philadelphia: Current Medicine, 2000:225, with permission.)

excessive aqueous humor flow results in very low IOP, shallow or flat chamber, and a prominently elevated bleb. Continued hypotony may result in serous choroidal detachment that further reduces aqueous humor production and worsens the situation. The surgeon should instruct the patient to avoid any activity that would cause his or her face to turn red and increase episcleral venous pressure. A large polymethyl methacrylate therapeutic contact lens, such as the Simmons lens, or a tight patch may be applied to diminish the flow of aqueous humor by increasing outflow resistance. If the chamber remains shallow but does not flatten, viscoelastic material may be injected into the anterior chamber to increase chamber depth and IOP. If the central anterior lens capsule and the corneal endothelium touch, then the anterior chamber should be reformed and choroidal detachment drained as soon as possible to minimize complications of cataract formation, corneal endothelial damage, anterior chamber inflammation, and bleb failure (9) (Figs. 8.7 and 8.8). Large choroidal detachments without corneal lenticular contact usually slowly resolve spontaneously without complication. However, extremely large choroidal detachments that touch one another in the central vitreous cavity ("kissing choroidal detachments") may lead to retinal surface complications. Patients with very shallow anterior

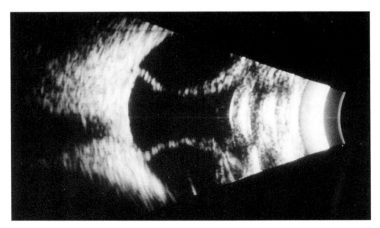

FIGURE 8.8. B-scan echography of large serous choroidal effusions of eye in Fig.8.7. (Reprinted from Parrish RK II, ed. *University of Miami Bascom Palmer Eye Institute Atlas of Ophthalmology.* Philadelphia: Current Medicine, 2000:226, with permission.)

chamber depth after trabeculectomy should be examined daily to determine if corneal–lenticular contact has developed.

Surgical Drainage of Choroidal Detachment

If the surgeon cannot identify the previously made paracentesis wound, a second paracentesis should be performed before proceeding. Frequently, the faint outline of the original tract can be identified following application of dilute fluorescein solution. The operative note should be reviewed to determine the location and orientation of the tract. Making a second paracentesis in a very soft eye with a flat anterior chamber is technically difficult; it is easier and safer to use the first one, if possible. The surgeon then injects BSS through a 27-gauge or 30-gauge cannula to deepen the anterior chamber and permit evaluation of flow into the bleb. BSS is replaced with viscoelastic material that raises IOP and maintains anterior chamber depth. Alternatively, an infusion cannula placed through the paracentesis tract can be used to maintain IOP. The assistant can control the flow of BSS and increase IOP to facilitate drainage of the detachment.

After deepening the anterior chamber, the surgeon places an inferior peripheral corneal traction suture near the 6:00 meridian and rotates the eye upward to expose the inferotemporal or inferonasal quadrant. Preoperative indirect ophthalmoscopy demonstrates the position and extent of the detachment. Usually the quadrant with the largest detachment is selected for the first drainage site. The surgeon makes a 3- to 4-mm radial conjunctival and Tenon's capsule incision, centered approximately 3 mm posterior to the limbus, with Westcott scissors (Storz Instruments, Bausch & Lomb, Rochester, NY) in the desired quadrant. Bleeding is controlled with light applications of cautery. A 3-mm radial scleral incision, positioned 3 mm posterior to the limbus, is outlined with a sharp blade (Fig. 8.9). The surgeon slowly and gently cuts through the scleral lamellae until the suprachoroidal space is reached. Darkening of the deepest part of the incision indicates that the remaining sclera is thin and suprachoroidal space is nearby. To improve visualization of the depth of the incision, the surgeon should grasp one incision lip with forceps using the nondominant hand while the assistant holds the other lip. With the dom-

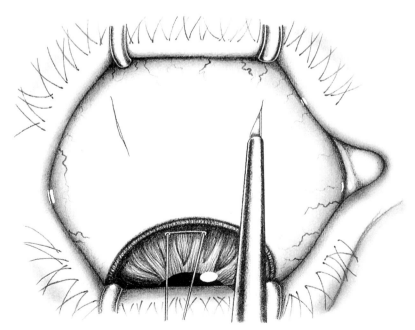

FIGURE 8.9. Drainage of choroidal effusion. Two inferiorly located sclerotomies minimize reformation of effusion.

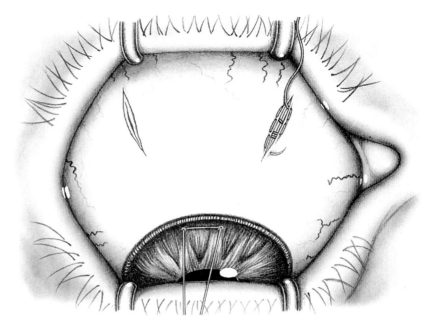

FIGURE 8.10. Drainage of choroidal effusion. Tenon's capsule and conjunctival closure over unsutured sclerotomies.

inant hand, the surgeon slowly cuts through the remaining scleral fibers. Upon entering the suprachoroidal space, yellow-tinged fluid spontaneously flows from the eye. Pressing the sclera while spreading the incision lips with a forceps facilitates drainage. Occasionally it may be necessary to introduce a spatula through the sclerotomy to gently press on the inner wall of the sclera to facilitate drainage.

We do not close the sclerotomies to facilitate postoperative drainage of the suprachoroidal effusion and to prevent reaccumulation. We close the conjunctiva and Tenon's

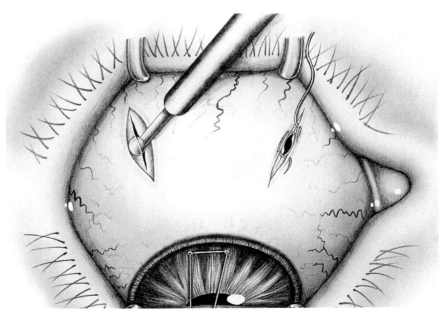

FIGURE 8.11. Drainage of choroidal effusion. Sclerectomies with a Kelly Descemet's punch (Storz Instruments, Bausch & Lomb, Rochester, NY) to produce 1.5-mm circular scleral openings.

capsule with a running 10-0 nylon suture (Fig. 8.10). Some surgeons use a Kelly Descemet's punch (Storz Instruments, Bausch & Lomb, Rochester, NY) to excise one or two fragments of the outer lip of the scleral incision before closing the conjunctiva (Fig. 8.11). After producing one drainage site, indirect ophthalmoscopy should be performed to determine the extent of residual detachment. If moderate detachments remain, then a similar procedure is performed in the other inferior quadrant. At the end of the procedure, the anterior chamber should be filled with BSS and the bleb and conjunctival wound inspected for any leakage that might have developed during the procedure. Occasionally an inferiorly located bleb may be seen in the immediate postoperative period that corresponds to the accumulation of serous fluid near the sclerotomy site.

SURGICAL PEARLS: SUTURELYSIS

- Do not perform suturelysis or massage if a conjunctival wound leak is identified.
- Always use a suturelysis lens to focus the laser energy.
- Cut the suture at its most posterior point of entry into the sclera. If the suture is cut in the middle, both ends can rotate superficially and perforate the conjunctiva.
- *To minimize hypotony, do not cut more than one suture per day.*
- *Do not cut a suture if you cannot examine the patient the following day.*
- Understand that complications associated with acutely lowered IOP, such as flat chamber, choroidal detachment, and delayed suprachoroidal hemorrhage, may rarely complicate argon laser suturelysis.

REFERENCES

1. Roth SM, Spaeth GL, Starita RJ, et al. The effects of postoperative corticosteroids on trabeculectomy and the clinical course of glaucoma: five-year follow-up study. *Ophth Surg* 1991;22:724–729.
2. Kolker AE. Visual prognosis in advanced glaucoma: a comparison of medical and surgical therapy for retention of vision in 101 eyes with advanced glaucoma. *Trans Am Ophthalmol Soc* 1977;75:539–555.
3. Traverso CE, Greenidge KC, Spaeth GL, et al. Focal pressure: a new method to encourage filtration after trabeculectomy. *Ophth Surg* 1984;15:62–65.
4. Hoskins HD Jr, Migliazzo C. Management of failing filtering blebs with the argon laser. *Ophth Surg* 1984; 15:731–733.
5. Savage JA, Condon GP, Lytle RA, et al. Laser suture lysis after trabeculectomy. *Ophthalmology* 1988;95:1631–1637.
6. Givens K, Shields MB. Suprachoroidal hemorrhage after glaucoma filtering surgery. *Am J Ophthalmol* 1987;103:689–694.
7. Liebmann JM, Weinreb RN, Ritch R. Angle-closure glaucoma associated with occult annular ciliary body detachment. *Arch Ophthalmol* 1998;116:731–735.
8. Shingleton BJ, Richter CU, Bellows AR, et al. Management of encapsulated filtration blebs. *Ophthalmology* 1990;97:63–68.
9. Dellaporta A. Scleral trephination for subchoroidal effusion. *Arch Ophthalmol* 1983;101:1917–1919.

WOUND HEALING MODULATION IN TRABECULECTOMY

5-Fluorouracil (5-FU) and mitomycin C (MMC) were first used to enhance bleb development after trabeculectomy in the early 1980s (1–9). Although the use of intraoperative topical MMC and postoperative subconjunctival 5-FU injections was initially limited to eyes whose conditions were associated with poor prognosis, recently these agents have been applied to eyes undergoing initial trabeculectomy (10,11). *The increased risks of late-onset endophthalmitis and bleb leaks associated with their use must be weighed against the benefits of intraocular pressure (IOP) control in eyes whose conditions are associated with a good prognosis (4–8).* Indications for use of these potent inhibitors of wound healing include aphakia and pseudophakia, history of failed filtering surgery, neovascular glaucoma (after panretinal photocoagulation), and African racial characteristics.

5-FLUOROURACIL

As initially described, 5-FU was given as a 5-mg subconjunctival injection (0.5 mL of a 10 mg/1.0 mL solution) twice daily on postoperative days 1 through 7 and once daily during postoperative days 8 through 14 after trabeculectomy (Fig. 9.1). The total dose, 105 mg, was frequently associated with the development of corneal or conjunctival

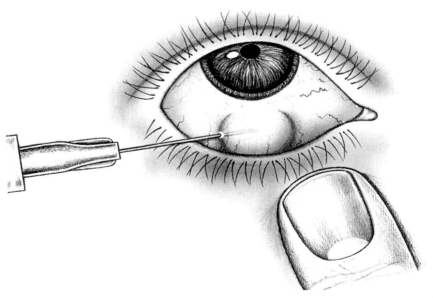

FIGURE 9.1. Postoperative subconjunctival injection of 5-fluorouracil administered 180 degrees from filtering site.

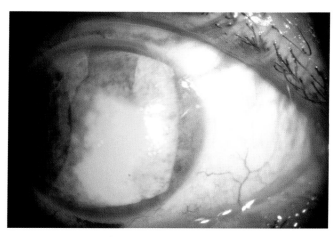

FIGURE 9.2. Corneal epithelial toxicity result from multiple postoperative subconjunctival injections of 5-fluorouracil.

epithelial defects or both, as well as persistent conjunctival wound leaks. Subconjunctival 5-FU should not be used in eyes with acquired limbal stem cell deficiency associated with alkali injury, drug-induced pseudopemphigoid, or aniridia. Eyes with corneal epithelial anterior basement membrane dystrophy and aqueous tear deficiency are at high risk to develop surface toxicity and persistent corneal epithelial defects (Fig 9.2).

Treatment has evolved to an intraoperative application of 5-FU on single or multiple cellulose sponge fragments, approximately 5 × 5 mm each, applied to the scleral surface and overlying subconjunctival tissue surrounding the filtering site (Fig. 9.3). The surgeon should apply the sponge soaked with the commercially available 5-FU solution (50 mg/mL, Adria Laboratories, Dublin, OH) before the flap is outlined to minimize the risk of intraocular penetration. The exposure duration is usually 3 to 5 minutes. Either a limbus- or a fornix-based conjunctival flap may be chosen; however, either incision must be

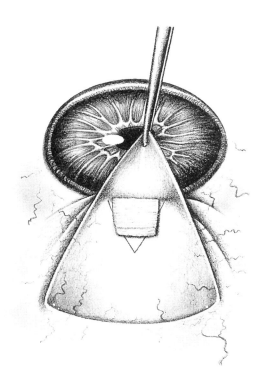

FIGURE 9.3. Intraoperative application of 5-fluorouracil or mitomycin C on cellulose sponge.

closed in a watertight fashion. Postoperative 5-mg subconjunctival injections (0.1 mL of a 50 mg/mL solution or 0.5 mL of a 10 mg/mL solution) are given in the quadrant adjacent to the bleb based on the appearance of the filtering site. To minimize discomfort, a cotton-tipped applicator soaked with proparacaine hydrochloride should be applied to the injection site for approximately 30 seconds. Clinical signs of early wound healing that are associated with bleb scarring, such as low bleb height, conjunctival bleb hyperemia, and lack of conjunctival epithelial edema (microcysts), are indications for beginning 5-FU injections. Injections are continued at every-other-day or every-third-day intervals until the vascularity is less prominent and microcysts are seen.

SURGICAL PEARLS FOR 5-FU USE

- Use commercially available 5-FU (50 mg/mL) for intraoperative application on cellulose sponge fragments.
- Absorb excess 5-FU with a dry cellulose sponges before irrigation.
- Irrigate the conjunctival surface with 20 mL of sterile saline solution after application.
- Inject postoperative 5-FU in the quadrant adjacent to or 180 degrees from bleb.
- Inject postoperative subconjunctival 5-FU, 5 mg (0.1 mL of 50 mg/mL solution).
- Apply proparacaine hydrochloride on cotton-tipped applicator over the injection site.
- Use a 30-gauge needle on tuberculin syringe to minimize leakage through the needle tract.

MITOMYCIN C

The application of MMC, a more potent inhibitor of fibroblast proliferation than 5-FU, results in the development of thin avascular blebs. MMC should be applied intraoperatively to the scleral surface in the same manner that was described for 5-FU. Care must be taken to avoid possible intraocular penetration of MMC, which can kill corneal endothelial cells. Reported concentrations and application durations have varied from 0.2 mg/mL to 0.5 mg/mL and from 2 to 5 minutes. Most surgeons use a 0.4 mg/mL concentration with an application duration of 3 to 4 minutes.

SURGICAL PEARLS FOR MITOMYCIN C USE

- Avoid contact between the edge of the conjunctival incision and MMC.
- Dissect the conjunctival and Tenon's capsule flap as one layer.
- Do not remove Tenon's capsule.
- Do not apply excessive pressure on the sponge by pulling the conjunctival flap posteriorly (limbus-based flap) or anteriorly (fornix-based flap). Doing so can cause squeezing of MMC from the sponge.
- Apply MMC prior to anterior chamber paracentesis or scleral flap dissection to minimize the risk of intraocular penetration.
- Dry the scleral surface with cellulose sponges to absorb excess MMC prior to irrigating with balanced sterile saline solution.

Several technical factors are important for the successful use of either 5-FU or MMC. Additional key points must be considered when planning argon laser suturelysis after 5-FU or MMC application.

SURGICAL PEARLS FOR TRABECULECTOMY TECHNIQUE AND ARGON SUTURELYSIS WITH 5-ANTIMETABOLITE USE

- Close limbus-based or fornix-based conjunctival flap in a watertight manner to avoid postoperative hypotony.
- Do not perform full-thickness surgery (trephination, thermal sclerostomy, posterior lip sclerectomy) with fornix-based flaps if use of MMC or 5-FU is anticipated.
- Use vascular tapered needles to close conjunctival incision (limbus based).
- Begin conjunctival closure during sponge application to save time.
- Consider argon laser suturelysis as a planned part of every trabeculectomy.
- To minimize the risk of hypotony associated with 5-FU or MMC use, never place fewer than three sutures in the scleral flap.
- Perform suturelysis if IOP is elevated and the bleb is flat by postoperative day 3 if neither 5-FU or MMC was used, by postoperative day 7 if 5-FU was used, and by postoperative day 14 if MMC was used. Most sutures are cut within the first 2 weeks, although suturelysis may be effective for up to 6 weeks or longer after MMC application.
- Delay suturelysis if possible until postoperative day 7 when the conjunctival wound is securely healed.
- Use short-duration (0.2 msec), low-power argon laser applications (300 mM) and small spot size (50 μm).
- Use either a Hoskins suturelysis lens or the four-mirror goniolens (see Fig. 8.3).
- Cut suture at the point of entry into the sclera at the location most posterior to the corneal–scleral junction. If the suture is cut in the middle, the cut ends may rotate superficially and perforate the overlying conjunctiva.
- *Never cut more than one suture per day.*
- *Avoid cutting a suture if you cannot examine the patient on the next day.*

REFERENCES

1. Weinreb RN. Adjusting the dose of 5-fluorouracil after filtration surgery to minimize side effects. *Ophthalmology* 1987;94:564–570.
2. Palmer SS. Mitomycin as adjunct chemotherapy with trabeculectomy. *Ophthalmology* 1991;98:317–321.
3. Stamper RL, McMenemy MG, Lieberman MF. Hypotonous maculopathy after trabeculectomy with subconjunctival 5-fluorouracil. *Am J Ophthalmol* 1992;114:544–553.
4. Parrish RK II. Who should receive antimetabolites after filtering surgery? *Arch Ophthalmol* 1992;110:1069–1071.
5. The Fluorouracil Filtering Surgery Study Group. Three-year follow-up of the Fluorouracil Filtering Surgery Study. *Am J Ophthalmol* 1993;115:82–92.
6. Katz GJ, Higginbotham EJ, Lichter PR, et al. Mitomycin C versus 5-fluorouracil in high-risk glaucoma filtering surgery; extended follow-up. *Ophthalmology* 1995;102:1263–1269.
7. Parrish R, Minckler D. "Late endophthalmitis": filtering surgery time bomb? *Ophthalmology* 1996;103:1167–1168.
8. The Fluorouracil Filtering Surgery Study Group. Five-year follow-up of the Fluorouracil Filtering Surgery Study. *Am J Ophthalmol* 1996;121:349–366.
9. Parrish RK II, Schiffman JC, Feuer WJ, et al. Prognosis and risk factors for early postoperative wound leaks after trabeculectomy with and without 5-fluorouracil. *Am J Ophthalmol* 2001;132:633–640.
10. Bindlish R, Condon GP, Schlosser JD, et al. Efficacy and safety of mitomycin-C in primary trabeculectomy; five year follow-up. *Ophthalmology* 2002;109:1336–1341.
11. Wu Dunn D, Cantor LB, Palanca-Capistrano AM, et al. A prospective randomized trial comparing intraoperative 5-fluorouracil versus mitomycin-C in primary trabeculectomy. *Am J Ophthalmol* 2002;134:521–528.

10

LATE COMPLICATIONS OF TRABECULECTOMY

Complications of trabeculectomy are not limited to the immediate postoperative period. Long-term changes in the bleb may predispose to leaks, blebitis, and endophthalmitis (1–5). Patients should understand the warning signs of early bleb infection so that urgent care can be sought. Late failure associated with bleb encapsulation may require revision if needling does not result in lowered intraocular pressure (IOP) (see Chapter 8).

LATE BLEB LEAKAGE

Thin-walled filtering blebs with few normal-appearing conjunctival blood vessels (ischemic blebs) associated with the use of 5-fluorouracil (5-FU) and mitomycin C (MMC) are at high risk to develop leaks (1) (Figs. 10.1 and 10.2). Leakage may not be apparent until the Seidel test has been performed. With small leaks, patients are usually asymptomatic and the eye is quiet with a normal or low IOP. The surgeon must decide whether to observe the leak, recommend medical treatment, or surgically intervene to close the leak. This decision is based on bleb location, history of conjunctivitis or prior bleb infection, patient compliance, and age. Patients with bleb leaks are at a higher risk of developing blebitis and endophthalmitis (1). After glaucoma filtering surgery, every patient should understand that simple "pink eye" or conjunctivitis may develop into a serious intraocular infection if not properly treated. *We advise these patients to immediately seek care for the following signs or symptoms: red eye (R), sensitivity to light (photophobia) (S), visual acuity change (V), and pain (P). The acronym RSVP is a helpful reminder to the patient.*

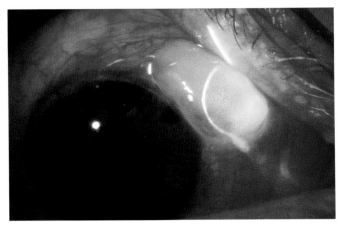

FIGURE 10.1. Thin avascular filtering bleb after trabeculectomy and intraoperative mitomycin C.

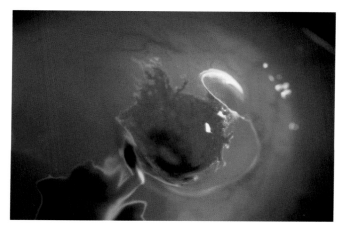

FIGURE 10.2. Seidel test of bleb in eye shown in Fig. 10.1.

Initially topical and oral glaucoma medications that reduce aqueous humor formation, such as beta blockers or carbonic anhydrase inhibitors, may be used to reduce the flow through the hole in the bleb wall. Although short-term topical antibiotics may be used, long-term use of broad-spectrum topical antibiotics should be avoided. The use of these drugs may eliminate the normal conjunctival flora and predispose to colonization with more virulent organisms.

AUTOLOGOUS BLOOD INJECTION

Autologous blood injection into the filtering bleb to promote wound healing has been advocated for the treatment for late-onset bleb leaks. After preparation of the antecubital fossa with topical povidone-iodine (Betadine) and isopropyl alcohol, an 18-gauge needle on a 3-mL syringe is used to withdraw blood from a large-caliber vein. After careful removal of 1 mL of whole blood, the needle is replaced with a sterile disposable 27-gauge needle. The needle tip is introduced through the conjunctiva, approximately 3 mm peripheral to the posterior bleb edge, and slowly advanced to the bleb wall where the blood is injected. If the blood enters the anterior chamber, a small hyphema may occur and temporarily reduce visual acuity. To minimize this complication, 0.1 to 0.2 mL of viscoelastic material introduced through a paracentesis tract may be placed at the fistula site prior to injection of blood. If the first bleb injection is not successful, the procedure may be repeated to further stimulate wound healing.

SURGICAL MANAGEMENT OF A LEAKING BLEB

If conservative measures fail to promote resolution of the bleb leak, surgical revision is the next option. Either conjunctival flap advancement, a technically easier procedure, or autologous conjunctival grafting usually stops the bleb leak (6–8).

Conjunctival Flap Advancement

Following placement of a clear corneal traction suture directly anterior to the leaking bleb, a temporal paracentesis tract is made. Viscoelastic material or balanced salt solution (BSS) is injected to maintain normal anterior chamber depth during the procedure (Fig. 10.3). A sharp blade is used to cut a small opening in the anterior conjunctival insertion adjacent to the bleb and the posterior blade of small blunt-tipped Westcott scissors (Storz Instruments, Bausch & Lomb, Rochester, NY) is passed into the subconjunctival space

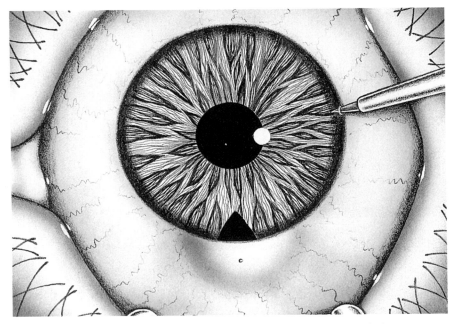

FIGURE 10.3. Conjunctival flap advancement. Paracentesis with sharp blade.

(Figs. 10.4 and Fig. 10.5). The surgeon cuts the posterior bleb margin free from the surrounding normal conjunctiva with the scissors and resects the superficial portion of the bleb. Care should be taken to remove all surface epithelium from the bleb surface and surrounding peripheral cornea with a sharp knife to enhance adherence of the conjunctival flap (Fig. 10.6). After blunt dissection with the scissor tips in the subconjunctival space, the conjunctival flap is grasped with serrated tissue forceps and pulled anteriorly to the limbus. The eye may be rotated in the direction of the bleb with the corneal traction

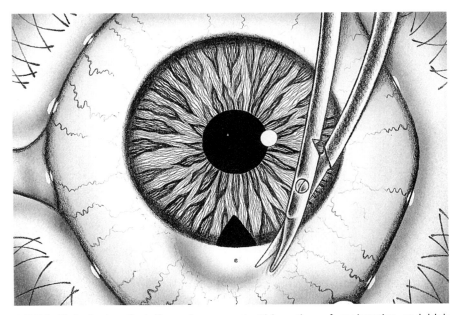

FIGURE 10.4. Conjunctival flap advancement. Disinsertion of conjunctiva and bleb excision.

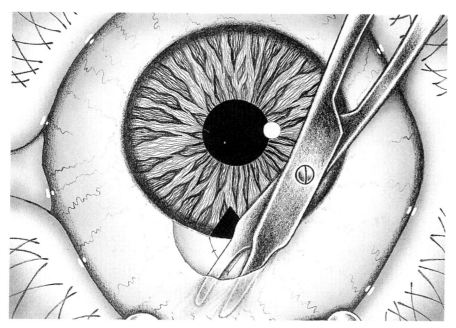

FIGURE 10.5. Conjunctival flap advancement. Dissection into sub-Tenon's space.

suture to increase conjunctival laxity and facilitate closure. If this maneuver does not improve conjunctival laxity, then a second and separate conjunctival incision, placed deeply in the fornix, may relax wound tension and permit the conjunctiva to slide anteriorly over the intact underlying Tenon's capsule. Care must be taken to avoid injuring the underlying superior rectus muscle. The conjunctiva is sutured to the anterior limbus with either multiple interrupted, horizontal mattress, or continuous running 10-0 nylon or 8-0 polyglactin sutures (Fig. 10.7). The surgeon injects BSS through the paracentesis tract to reform the bleb and check for wound leaks (Fig. 10.8).

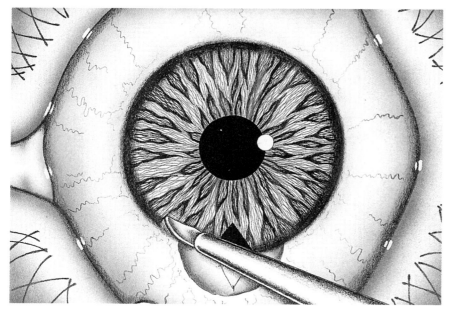

FIGURE 10.6. Conjunctival flap advancement. Removal of limbal and peripheral corneal epithelium.

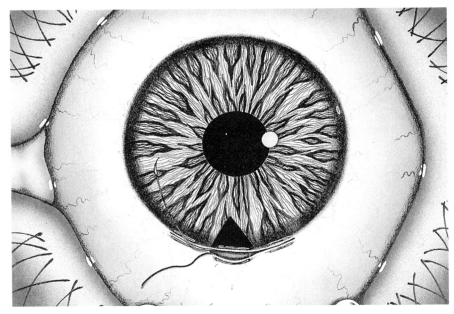

FIGURE 10.7. Conjunctival flap advancement. Wound closure with multiple horizontal mattress sutures.

Conjunctival Free Graft

If conjunctival advancement is unlikely to cover the area of a large avascular bleb after resection, an autologous free conjunctival graft is used. After positioning the lid speculum and placing a corneal traction suture, a paracentesis tract is made and viscoelastic is injected (Fig. 10.9). The size of the bleb to be resected is measured and a free conjunctiva graft, approximately 1 to 2 mm wider and longer than the bleb, is outlined. Two 8-0 Vicryl sutures (Ethicon Products Worldwide, Johnson & Johnson, Somerville, NJ) are placed at each corner near the limbus to orient the graft (Fig. 10.10). Methylene blue can

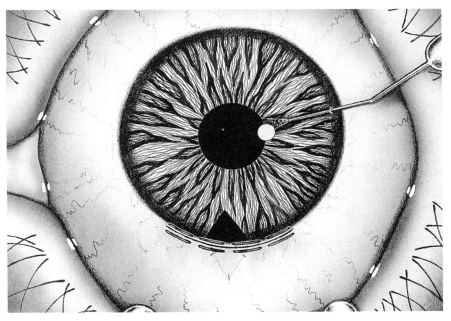

FIGURE 10.8. Conjunctival flap advancement. Balanced salt solution injection to elevate bleb and inspect for watertight wound closure.

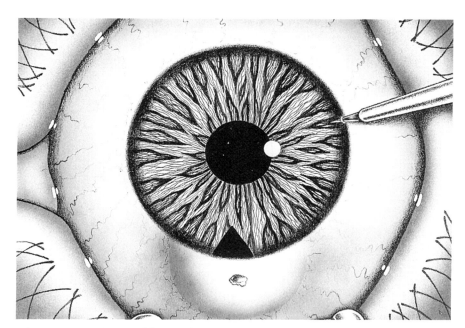

FIGURE 10.9. Conjunctival free graft. Paracentesis with sharp blade.

be used to paint the anterior superficial surface to assist in maintaining the correct orientation of the graft. After harvesting of the graft, the donor site wound is closed (Fig. 10.11). Following resection of the avascular bleb, normal vascularized conjunctiva will be present at the wound margins (Fig. 10.12). The free graft is positioned to ensure the correct orientation with the epithelial side facing upward and the limbal side toward the

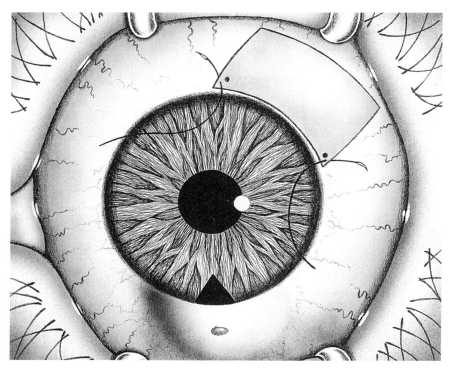

FIGURE 10.10. Conjunctival free graft. Harvesting donor conjunctival graft from inferior conjunctiva.

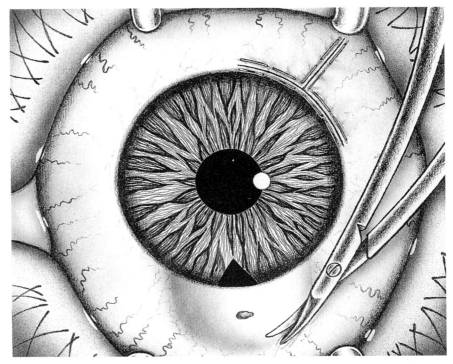

FIGURE 10.11. Conjunctival free graft. Donor wound closure and resection of leaking bleb.

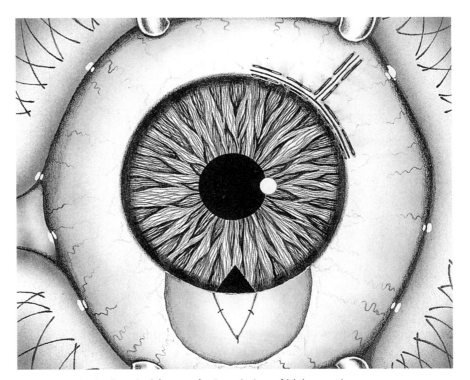

FIGURE 10.12. Conjunctival free graft. Completion of bleb resection.

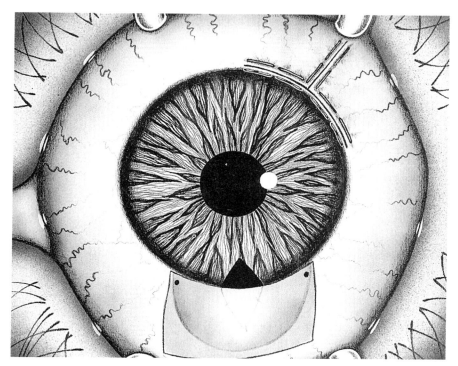

FIGURE 10.13. Conjunctival free graft. Donor graft in conjunctival host bed.

cornea (Fig. 10.13). To facilitate this, Vicryl sutures are left in the graft. Finally the graft is sutured with four interrupted sutures in the corners of the graft and a running suture passing through the rest of the graft; or with interrupted mattress sutures. The wound is inspected with a dry cellulose sponge following injection of BSS through the paracentesis (Fig. 10.14).

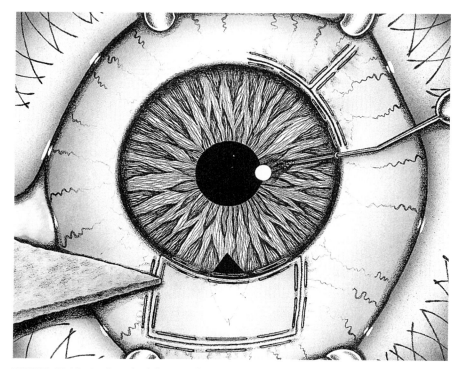

FIGURE 10.14. Conjunctival free graft. Inspection of graft after injection of balanced salt solution into anterior chamber.

SURGICAL REVISION OF ENCAPSULATED BLEBS

If bleb needling does not result in sufficiently lowered IOP, surgical bleb revision is recommended. After positioning a lid speculum and applying topical anesthesia, a paracentesis tract is made. The original limbus-based conjunctival incision is opened and the anterior conjunctiva is carefully dissected from the underlying cyst wall with blunt-tipped scissors. After elevation and separation of the conjunctiva to the point of its limbal attachment, a portion of the cyst wall is excised with Vannas scissors (Storz Instruments, Bausch & Lomb, Rochester, NY) (Fig. 10.15). After closing the incision, BSS, injected through the paracentesis, is used to reform the anterior chamber and check the wound closure. 5-FU on a cellulose sponge fragment may be applied to the cyst wall and the subconjunctival surface to reduce further scarring (see Chapter 9). *5-FU should not be applied after removal of the cyst wall.*

LATE POSTOPERATIVE INFECTION

Infection after trabeculectomy is a greater concern in the late postoperative period than immediately after surgery. Bacterial proliferation may be localized in the bleb ("blebitis") or invade the eye to produce endophthalmitis. The increasing use of 5-FU and MMC has resulted in a higher prevalence of thin and ischemic blebs that are more likely to become infected.

Clinical Features

Patient with blebitis may complain of redness, sensitivity to light, blurred vision, foreign body sensation, tearing, and mild discharge. The infected bleb stands out as a white circular zone against the diffusely hyperemic background. ("white over red" sign) (Fig. 10.16). The IOP is usually normal or low, and the Seidel test may be positive (Fig. 10.17). The anterior chamber may demonstrate mild to moderate flare and cellular response. *Severe pain, marked loss of vision, and hypopyon indicate that blebitis has progressed to endophthalmitis and treatment should include intravitreal antibiotics.* After dilation the vitreous should be carefully examined for the presence of cellular infiltration. Involvement of the vitreous is diagnostic for endophthalmitis.

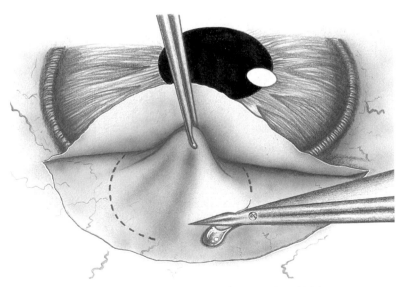

FIGURE 10.15. Surgical revision of encapsulated bleb.

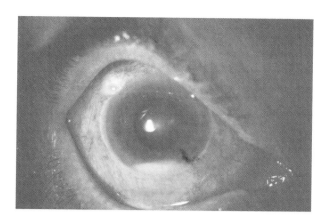

FIGURE 10.16. "White on red" sign of blebitis and hypopyon formation of endophthalmitis.

Risk Factors

The following risk factors have been identified for late-onset infection after glaucoma filtering surgery: inferior location of the bleb (4:00 to 8:00), chronic bleb leakage, 5-FU and MMC use. Recurrent bacterial posterior marginal blepharitis, contact lens use, and immunosuppression may also predispose to infection. Recent upper respiratory tract infection with *Haemophilus influenzae* associated with involvement of multiple mucous membrane surfaces may also precede blebitis and present as a severe tracheobronchitis with bilateral conjunctivitis.

Diagnosis

Cultures should be taken of the bleb surface and the eyelid margin before beginning antibiotic therapy. If endophthalmitis is suspected, then anterior chamber and vitreous taps should also be performed.

Management of Blebitis

Although blebitis is usually treated empirically before culture results are available, subsequent therapy should be changed based on the clinical outcome and the culture results. Topical treatment with fortified antibiotics is the mainstay of therapy, although subconjunctival injections are given if topical administration is not possible. Oral antibiotics are infrequently

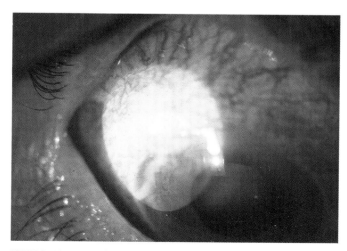

FIGURE 10.17. Seidel test over thin superior bleb with marked leakage of aqueous humor. (Same eye as in Fig. 10.16.)

used as bactericidal concentrations are obtained with topical therapy. After beginning therapy patients should be monitored for change in the status of their vision and ocular pain within 12 hours. Topical corticosteroids may reduce inflammation in the bleb but should be used only after the infection has been eradicated. If pain or intraocular inflammation worsens during treatment with topical antibiotics, then anterior chamber and vitreous taps should be performed and intravitreal antibiotics given for presumed endophthalmitis.

Topical Antibiotics

- Fortified vancomycin (50 mg/mL) and fortified gentamicin (14 mg/mL) or fortified tobramycin (14 mg/mL) alternating every 2 hours until improvement is seen.
- Topical fluoroquinolones may be used initially although they do not adequately treat gram-positive microorganisms, such as *Streptococcus* species.

Subconjunctival Dosages

- Vancomycin: 25 mg/0.5 mL.
- Ceftazidime: 50 mg/0.5 mL.

Oral

- Ofloxacin 200 to 400 mg twice a day, or ciprofloxacin 250 to 750 mg twice a day.

Management of Endophthalmitis

Endophthalmitis is managed with intravitreal antibiotics after vitreous cultures have been taken (tap and inject) with or without pars plana vitrectomy. As with blebitis, initial broad-spectrum antibiotic treatment is altered depending on the clinical outcome and the results of smears and cultures. The patient should be examined 12 to 24 hours after beginning treatment to evaluate the effectiveness of treatment.

After performing a vitreous tap or a pars plana vitrectomy, smears and cultures are taken, and antibiotics are injected.

Intravitreal Injection

- Ceftazidime 2.25 mg/0.1 mL or amikacin 400 µg/0.1 mL.
- Vancomycin 1.0 mg/0.1 mL.
- If corticosteroids given, 400 µg/0.1 mL dexamethasone is administered.

REFERENCES

1. Jampel HD, Quigley HA, Kerrigan-Baumrind LA, et al. Risk factors for late-onset infection following glaucoma filtration surgery. *Arch Ophthalmol* 2001;119:1001-1008.
2. Chen PP, Gedde SJ, Budenz DL, Parrish RK II. Outpatient treatment of bleb infection. *Arch Ophthalmol* 1997;115:1124–1128.
3. Ciulla TA, Beck AD, Topping TM, Baker AS. Blebitis, early endophthalmitis, and late endophthalmitis after glaucoma-filtering surgery. *Ophthalmology* 1997;104:986–995.
4. DeBry PW, Perkins TW, Heatley G, et al. Incidence of late-onset bleb-related complications following trabeculectomy with mitomycin. *Arch Ophthalmol* 2002;120:297–300.
5. Kangas TA, Greenfield DS, Flynn HW Jr, et al. Delayed-onset endophthalmitis associated with conjunctival filtering blebs. *Ophthalmology* 1997;104:746–752.
6. Sugar HS: Complications, repair and reoperation of antiglaucoma filtering blebs. *Am J Ophthalmol* 1967;63:825–833.
7. Burnstein AL, WuDunn D, Knotts SL, et al. Conjunctival advancement versus non-incisional treatment for late-onset glaucoma filtering bleb leaks. *Ophthalmology* 2002;109:71–75.
8. Myers JS, Yang CB, Herndon LW, et al. Excisional bleb revision to correct overfiltration or leakage. *J Glaucoma* 2000;9:169–173.

11

CATARACT AND GLAUCOMA: COMBINED PROCEDURES

Glaucoma and cataract, two common ocular conditions, often coexist in older patients. Treatment should be individualized according to the severity of glaucomatous damage, intraocular pressure (IOP) level, and visual disability related to the cataract (1–4).

TECHNIQUES AND ALTERNATIVES

Three surgical options may be pursued in the management of patients with cataract and glaucoma:

- Cataract extraction/intraocular lens (IOL) implantation with continued medical glaucoma therapy or subsequent trabeculectomy, if necessary
- Trabeculectomy alone and subsequent cataract extraction
- Combined cataract extraction/IOL and trabeculectomy as a single procedure

The first option, cataract extraction/IOL without trabeculectomy, is performed when the cataract accounts for the decreased visual acuity, glaucomatous damage is mild, and IOP is easily controlled. With advanced glaucomatous damage and uncontrolled IOP on maximal medical therapy, we usually prefer the second option, trabeculectomy and subsequent cataract extraction, preferably after 6 months. We perform combined cataract and glaucoma surgery in patients with visually disabling cataracts and marginally controlled IOP and in those who are poorly compliant with medical therapy. Combined phacoemulsification cataract extraction/IOL implantation and trabeculectomy with the intraoperative application of mitomycin C or 5-fluorouracil has become increasing popular (2).

We describe two combined cataract and glaucoma operations, phacoemulsification or extracapsular extraction, combined with trabeculectomy.

PREOPERATIVE MEDICATION: ANESTHESIA

Phacoemulsification and trabeculectomy (phacotrabeculectomy) may be performed under topical anesthesia in the cooperative patient. Miotics should be discontinued for at least a week, and 2 hours before surgery the pupil should be widely dilated with 1% cyclopentolate hydrochloride and 2.5% phenylephrine hydrochloride applied every 15 minutes. Additional topical nonsteroidal anti-inflammatory drops, such as 0.5% ketorolac tromethamine (Acular, Allergan, Irvine, CA), 0.1% diclofenac sodium (Voltaren, Ciba Vision, Duluth, GA), or 0.03% flurbiprofen sodium (Bausch & Lomb Pharmaceutical, Tampa, FL), may prolong intraoperative pupillary dilation. If the surgeon chooses the retrobulbar route, we suggest using a blunt-tipped cannula to inject the anesthetic agents through a small inferotemporal conjunctival incision to minimize periorbital bleeding.

PHACOTRABECULECTOMY

Phacotrabeculectomy may be performed with one incision for both the phacoemulsification and the trabeculectomy (one site) or with two separate incisions (two sites). Although one-site surgery requires less operative time, two-site procedures may have the advantage of placing the filtering site, usually located at the 12:00 position, distant to the temporal clear corneal incision. When performing two-site surgery, we prefer dissecting the trabeculectomy flap at the superior limbus before entering the anterior chamber and then completing phacoemulsification through a separate corneal incision. After completing the cataract extraction/IOL implantation, the surgeon returns to the superior surgical site, removes the inner block, and completes the trabeculectomy.

SINGLE-INCISION COMBINED SURGERY

Traction Suture

In a cooperative patient with topical anesthesia, a clear cornea traction suture is usually not necessary. With retrobulbar, peribulbar, or general anesthesia, we use a traction suture (see Chapter 5).

Conjunctival Incision

Either a limbus-based or a fornix-based peritomy can be used for one-site surgery (see Chapter 5).

Cauterization

Light cauterization controls bleeding without damaging the overlying conjunctiva. We prefer a blunt-tipped bipolar diathermy (Bipolar Instrument 18-Gauge Straight, Medtronic, Jacksonville, FL) to minimize thermal injury.

Paracentesis

The paracentesis may be made before or after dissection of the scleral tunnel. Filling the anterior chamber with either saline or viscoelastic material increases IOP and facilitates scleral tunnel dissection. If the surgeon inadvertently enters the anterior chamber more posteriorly than planned, he can redirect the incision angle more safely when the chamber depth is maintained with viscoelastic material. Intracameral acetylcholine, anesthetics, and auxiliary instruments may be introduced through the tract during phacoemulsification. A sharp blade or a 21-gauge needle may be used to make the tract (Fig. 11.1). A second paracentesis is needed if the surgeon prefers bimanual cortical lens removal. The anterior chamber should be filled with balanced salt solution (BSS), or viscoelastic before performing a second paracentesis.

Phacoemulsification Incision

The superiorly located scleral tunnel incision is performed in three steps. The first cut, a straight half-thickness 3.5 mm scleral groove that straddles the 12:00 meridian, is made with a sharp blade approximately 2.5 mm posterior to the limbus (Fig. 11.2). The second incision, a 3.5-mm-wide scleral–corneal tunnel, is dissected approximately 1 mm into the peripheral clear cornea with a crescent knife (Fig. 11.3). The third incision that enters the anterior chamber is made through an oblique incision at the most anterior point of the tunnel with a keratome (Fig. 11.4). The surgeon upon seeing the keratome tip in the anterior chamber redirects the blade angle parallel to the iris and advances it at the midante-

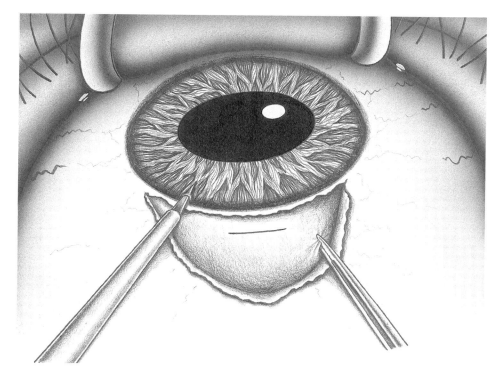

FIGURE 11.1. Phacotrabeculectomy. Paracentesis with sharp blade for second instrument and anterior chamber reformation.

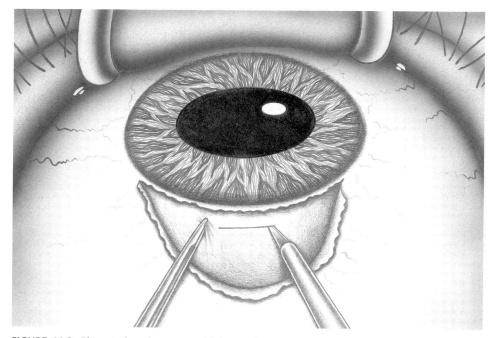

FIGURE 11.2. Phacotrabeculectomy. Initial straight 3.5-mm vertical incision, 2.5 mm posterior to the limbus.

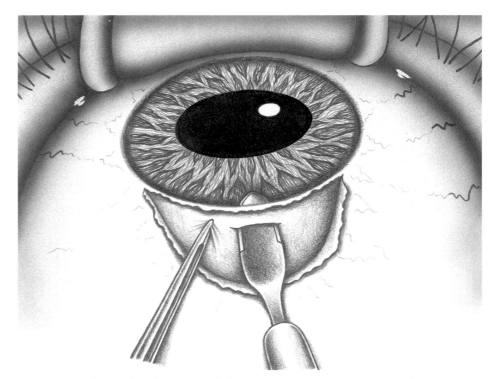

FIGURE 11.3. Phacotrabeculectomy. Limbal tunnel dissection with crescent knife into peripheral clear cornea, the width of the incision.

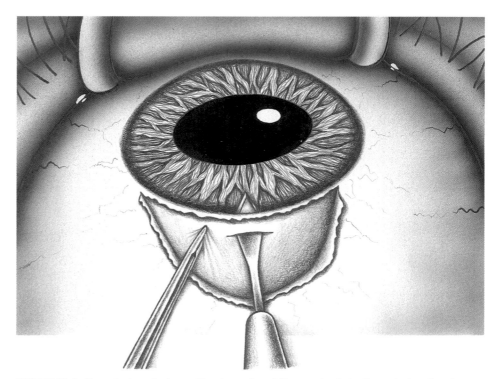

FIGURE 11.4. Phacotrabeculectomy. Keratome for oblique entry into the anterior chamber.

rior chamber plane. Failure to redirect the blade angle may result in inadvertent perforation of the anterior lens capsule.

The Small Pupil

Long-term miotic therapy or pseudoexfoliation syndrome or both may prevent sufficient pupillary dilation required for safe phacoemulsification. We prefer manipulating the pupil to achieve a diameter of at least 5 mm before beginning lens removal. This may result in a permanently dilated and poorly reactive pupil. The patient should be counseled regarding this possibility before surgery.

Stretching the pupil with two Kuglen hooks usually produces adequate pupillary enlargement. After filling the anterior chamber with a viscoelastic material, the surgeon introduces one Kuglen iris hook through the tunnel incision and a second Kuglen hook through the paracentesis incision. The inferior and superior pupillary borders near the 6 and 12 o'clock meridian are engaged with the hooks that are oriented in opposite directions. The surgeon slowly stretches the pupil by pushing each hook toward the chamber angle. The maneuver is repeated at the 3 and 9 o'clock meridians. After this maneuver, the anterior chamber is filled with additional viscoelastic material to further enlarge the pupil. Stretching occasionally causes minimal iris bleeding at the pupillary border that spontaneously stops.

If stretching does not result in adequate dilation, the surgeon may either perform multiple 0.5-mm radial sphincterotomies with Vannas scissors or place four iris hooks through 27-gauge corneal stab incisions at the 1:00. 5:00, 7:00, and 11:00 positions to enlarge the pupil. *The angle of the stab wounds adjacent to the phacoemulsification incision should be made parallel to the iris plane to minimize tenting of the peripheral iris toward the phacoemulsification hand piece entry site.* The surgeon should anticipate more postoperative inflammation than usual if pupillary manipulation is required.

Capsulotomy

A continuous circular capsulorrhexis, performed with a Utrata forceps (Katena Products, Inc., Denville, NJ) under viscoelastic material, is our preferred technique. After puncturing the paracentral anterior lens capsule and raising a flap with the lateral motion of a cystotome, the flap is grasped and rotated in a circular fashion to complete the capsulorrhexis (Figs. 11.5 and 11.6).

To safely perform a capsulorrhexis, the anterior chamber must remain formed and filled with viscoelastic material to maintain a clear view. Frequent regrasping of the capsular flap near its point of insertion with the untorn capsule and directing the tear toward the center of the pupil helps the surgeon control the capsulotomy size. Capsulotomies larger than 7 mm may disrupt the central zonular insertion.

Hydrodissection and Hydrodelamination

The surgeon injects BSS through a 27-gauge cannula under the anterior lens capsule with a 5- mL syringe until he sees a fluid wave pass behind the nucleus (hydrodissection; Fig. 11.7). To better outline the nuclear boundary, he may inject additional BSS at the level of the cortex centrally toward the nucleus to produce a "golden ring" (hydrodelamination). A freely mobile nucleus within the capsular bag and an intact continuous curvilinear capsulorrhexis simplify the procedure and promote safe phacoemulsification.

Phacoemulsification

Many techniques, such as Chip and Flip, Crack and Flip, Phaco Chop, Stop and Chop, and Divide and Conquer have been described. These procedures may be performed in the anterior chamber, at the iris plane, or within the capsular bag (3). We prefer the

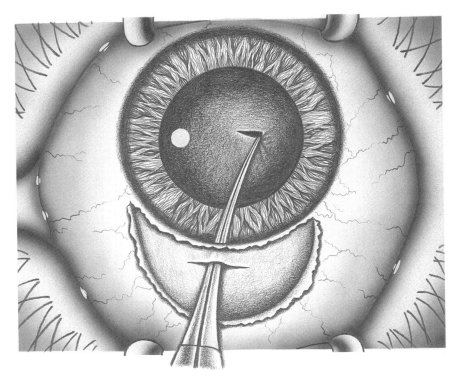

FIGURE 11.5. Phacotrabeculectomy. Initial anterior capsular perforation with the Utrata forceps (Katena Products, Inc., Denville, NJ) tips begins the capsulorrhexis.

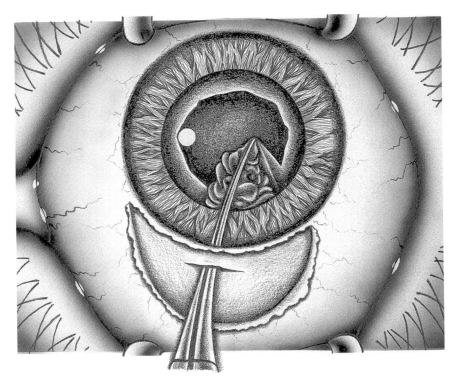

FIGURE 11.6. Phacotrabeculectomy. Completion of continuous circular capsulorrhexis with Utrata forceps.

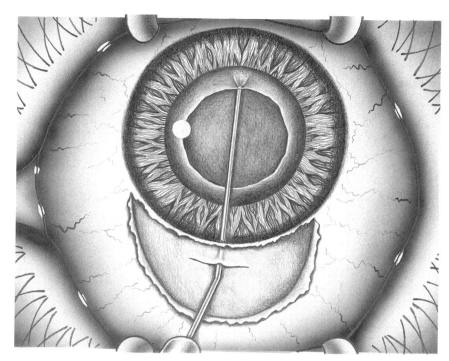

FIGURE 11.7. Phacotrabeculectomy. Hydrodissection of balanced salt solution under the anterior capsular edge.

"divide and conquer" technique, in which the nucleus is divided into four equally sized pieces and each is emulsified separately within the capsular bag (Figs. 11.8, 11.9, and 11.10).

Cortex Removal

The surgeon uses a standard dual-function irrigation and aspiration handpiece to remove cortex beginning at the 6 o'clock and ending at the 12 o'clock position (Fig. 11.11). Bimanual removal with aspiration and irrigation through separate sites simplifies removal of subincisional cortex, particularly with poor pupillary dilation.

Intraocular Lens Implantation

The surgeon enlarges the tunnel width depending on the IOL chosen. After filling the anterior chamber with viscoelastic material and introducing the IOL in the bag (Fig. 11.12), the viscoelastic material is removed and the pupil is pharmacologically constricted. Attention is now turned to completion of the trabeculectomy.

Trabeculectomy

Although we prefer excising the inner block with a Kelly Descemet's punch (Storz Instruments, Bausch & Lomb, Rochester, NY), Vannas scissors may also be used (Figs. 11.13 and 11.14). The surgeon may pass the punch through the tunnel without enlarging the incision or make one or two cuts at the tunnel edge, to form a triangular or rectangular scleral flap, respectively. The tunnel edge cuts improve visualization of the scleral bed. After inner block removal, a peripheral iridectomy is completed as previously described (see Chapter 5).

(text continues on page 101)

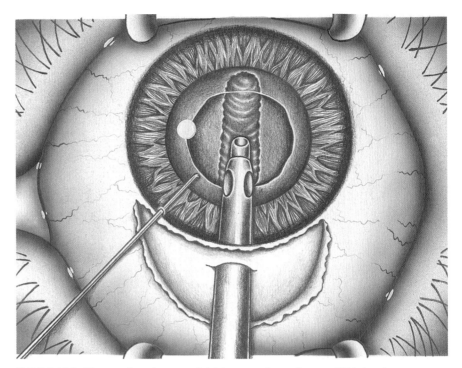

FIGURE 11.8. Phacotrabeculectomy. Initial groove in nucleus to 80% depth.

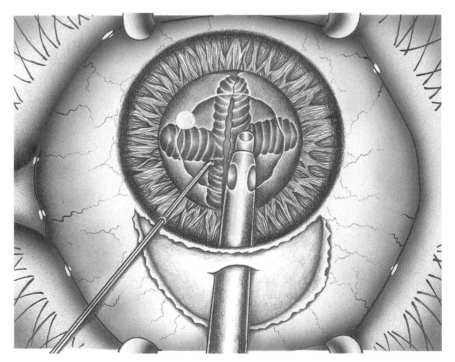

FIGURE 11.9. Phacotrabeculectomy. Cracking of nucleus into quadrants with phaco probe and second instrument.

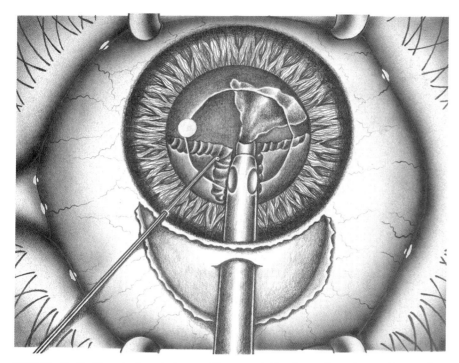

FIGURE 11.10. Phacotrabeculectomy. Phacoemulsification of each quadrant after nuclear cracking.

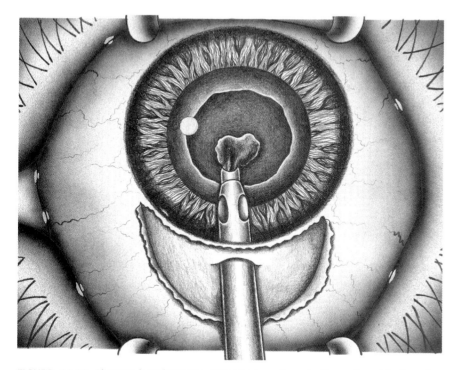

FIGURE 11.11. Phacotrabeculectomy. Irrigation and aspiration of residual cortex under direct visualization.

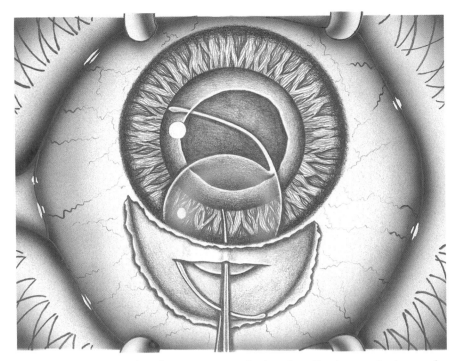

FIGURE 11.12. Phacotrabeculectomy. Intraocular lens insertion in capsular bag under viscoelastic cover.

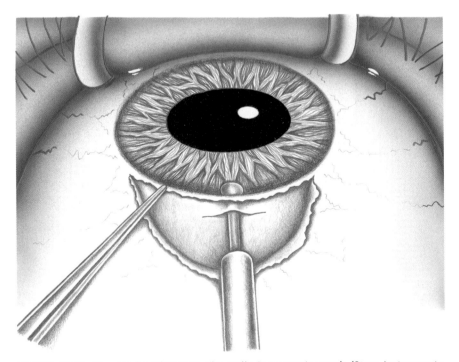

FIGURE 11.13. Phacotrabeculectomy. The Kelly Descemet's punch (Storz Instruments, Bausch & Lomb, Rochester, NY) positioned anterior to the scleral spur.

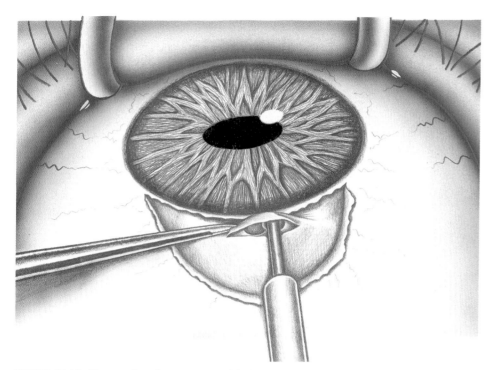

FIGURE 11.14. Phacotrabeculectomy. Inner block removal with Kelly Descemet's punch (Storz Instruments, Bausch & Lomb, Rochester, NY).

Closure of the Scleral Flap

If one edge of the scleral tunnel was cut, the corner should be closed with a single 10-0 nylon suture and the knot buried. If two cuts were made to produce a standard rectangular scleral flap, one suture should be placed at each corner. Additional sutures are placed as needed to adjust the outflow. The surgeon judges the rate of aqueous outflow by injecting BSS through the paracentesis tract and checking the flap for leakage with a dry cellulose sponge (Fig. 11.15).

Conjunctiva Closure and End of the Procedure

Conjunctival closure in phacotrabeculectomy is identical to that for standard trabeculectomy (see Chapter 5). To evaluate wound closure, the surgeon wipes the incision with a cellulose sponge while injecting BSS through the paracentesis (Fig. 11.16). As prolonged dilatation may lead to pupillary IOL capture, atropine should not be instilled.

EXTRACAPSULAR CATARACT EXTRACTION COMBINED WITH TRABECULECTOMY

Indications for combined extracapsular cataract extraction (ECCE) and trabeculectomy are similar to phacotrabeculectomy. Unavailability of phacoemulsification equipment, increased nucleus brunescence, reduced endothelial cell density, and Morgagni's cataracts are factors that favor extracapsular technique rather than phacoemulsification.

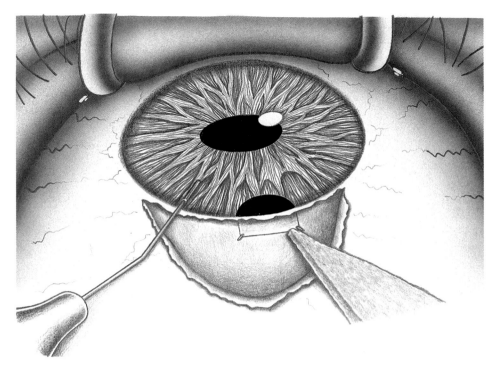

FIGURE 11.15. Phacotrabeculectomy. Assessment of filtration through the scleral flap with cellulose sponge as balanced salt solution is injected through paracentesis tract.

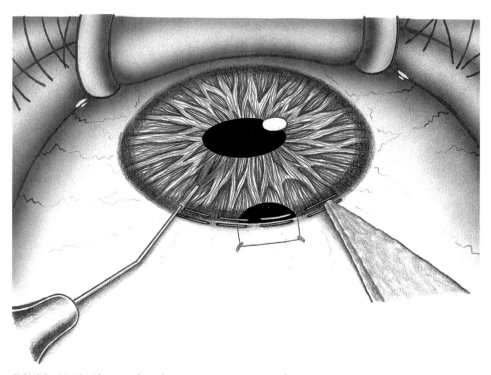

FIGURE 11.16. Phacotrabeculectomy. Assessment of conjunctival closure with cellulose sponge as balanced salt solution is injected through paracentesis tract.

Cataract and Glaucoma: Combined Procedures

Anesthesia

Peribulbar anesthetics, approximately 3 mL of a 1:4 mixture of 2% or 4% lidocaine hydrochloride and 0.75% bupivacaine hydrochloride, are injected in the inferotemporal quadrant. A supplemental 2-mL injection may be given in the superonasal quadrant, if necessary.

Peritomy

To perform a fornix-based peritomy, the surgeon grasps the conjunctiva with non-toothed forceps, just posterior to its insertion and cuts a 3-mm incision with micro Westcott scissors (Storz Instruments, Bausch & Lomb, Rochester, NY) at the anterior limbus. With the scissors held tangentially to the limbus, the posterior scissors blade is introduced through the incision and the conjunctival is disinserted from the 10:00 to the 2:00 meridian. Light cautery is used for conjunctiva and episcleral hemostasis. The conjunctiva should be moistened with BSS throughout the procedure to prevent drying and possible tearing.

Scleral Incision

While fixing the eye with 0.12-mm Castroviejo forceps (Katena Products, Inc., Denville, NJ), the surgeon cuts a 50% thickness 10-mm limbal groove approximately 2 mm posterior to the conjunctival insertion with a sharp round-tip blade. If the surgeon is right handed, the incision is most easily directed from the surgeon's left to the right, and in the opposite direction for the left-handed surgeon. The path of incision deviates 2 mm posteriorly from the 11:00 to the 1:00 meridian. (Fig. 11.17). A crescent knife is used to dissect the central scleral flap and the remainder of the incision 1 mm into clear peripheral cornea (Fig. 11.18). The surgeon enters the anterior chamber with a keratome to produce a three-step incision (Fig. 11.19).

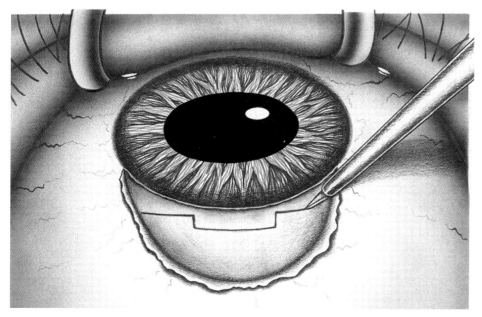

FIGURE 11.17. Extracapsular cataract extraction combined with trabeculectomy. Initial 10-mm partial thickness incision located 2 mm posterior to the limbus. Note that the middle 3 mm of the incision deviates posteriorly to form the trabeculectomy flap.

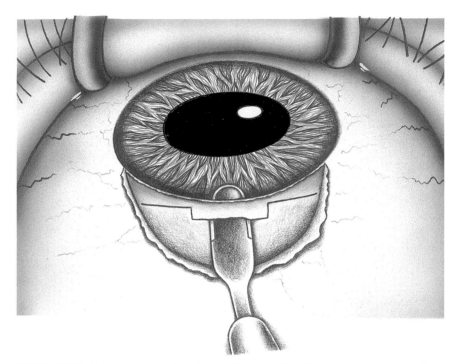

FIGURE 11.18. Extracapsular cataract extraction combined with trabeculectomy. Crescent knife dissection into peripheral clear cornea along entire incision length.

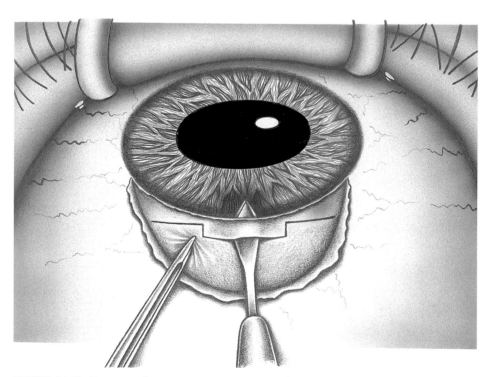

FIGURE 11.19. Extracapsular cataract extraction combined with trabeculectomy. Anterior chamber entry at oblique angle.

Capsulotomy

A 6-mm continuous circular capsulorrhexis, slightly larger than that used for phacoemulsification, is made as described above. The tip of the Utrata forceps or cystotome is used to begin the tear in the paracentral part of the anterior lens capsule (Fig. 11.20). If necessary, multiple relaxing incisions may be made in the capsulotomy to facilitate nuclear dissection.

Hydrodissection

Hydrodissection and hydrodelamination are performed as described previously (Figs. 11.21 and 11.22). These important maneuvers make safe removal of the nucleus possible.

Enlargement of the Scleral Wound

The surgeon uses a keratome or a sharp blade to fashion a valved 10-mm incision.

Removal of the Nucleus

Two techniques may be used to safely remove the nucleus. In the first, the surgeon uses a cystotome to cut the anterior lens capsule at the 10:00, 12:00, and 2:00 meridians after filling the anterior chamber with viscoelastic material. By applying light pressure 2 mm posteriorly to the incision with a closed 0.12 forceps and additional force at the 6:00 meridian, the superior pole of the nucleus usually prolapses into the anterior chamber superficial to the iris plane. Continued depression on the superior wound lip permits the nucleus to slide through the incision.

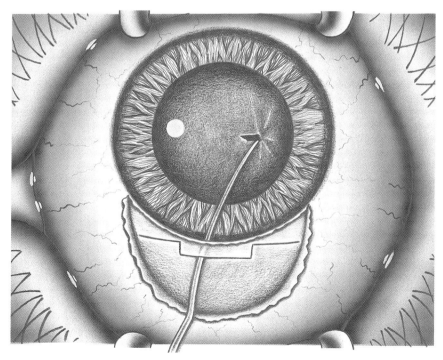

FIGURE 11.20. Extracapsular cataract extraction combined with trabeculectomy. Anterior capsular perforation with Utrata forceps or cystotome to begin capsulorrhexis.

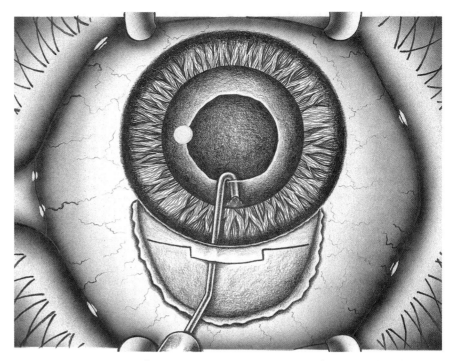

FIGURE 11.21. Extracapsular cataract extraction combined with trabeculectomy. Hydrodissection with balanced salt solution at 12 o'clock position with J-shape cannula.

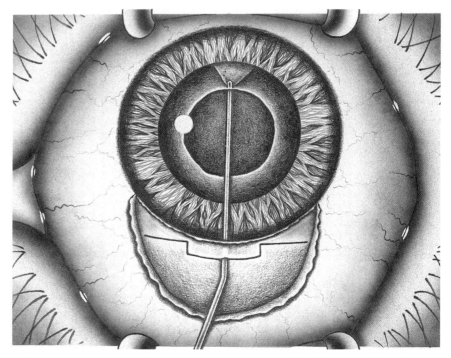

FIGURE 11.22. Extracapsular cataract extraction combined with trabeculectomy. Hydrodelamination with straight 26-gauge cannula tip under anterior capsule directed to the nucleus.

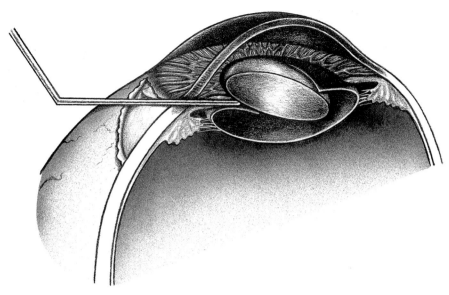

FIGURE 11.23. Extracapsular cataract extraction combined with trabeculectomy. A 26-gauge cannula positioned under the superior nuclear pole and injection of balanced salt solution to prolapse the nucleus anteriorly.

For the second technique, a 26-gauge cannula is used to carefully inject BSS under the capsulotomy edge at the 12:00 meridian, until the superior pole of the nucleus prolapses out of the capsular bag (Fig. 11.23). The nucleus is then rotated out of the bag with the cannula or cystotome, through the capsulotomy into the anterior chamber. An irrigating vectis is gently placed under the nucleus and BSS is gently injected at the 6:00 meridian to deliver the nucleus through the incision (Fig. 11.24).

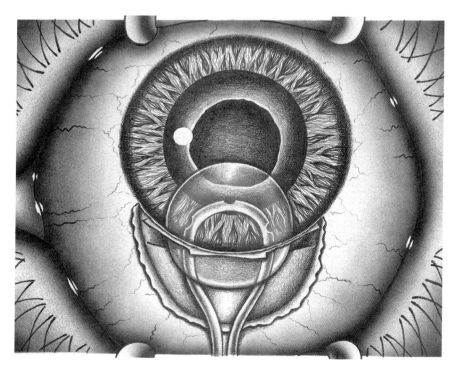

FIGURE 11.24. Extracapsular cataract extraction combined with trabeculectomy. An irrigating vectis for delivery of nucleus.

Cortex Removal

The surgeon may use a dual-function automated removal system or a manual technique, such as with the combined irrigation and aspiration Simcoe style cannula (Katena Products, Inc., Denville, NJ). Alternatively, a separate incision may be used for irrigation and aspiration. If the cataract wound is sufficiently beveled, it may not be necessary to close the incision before proceeding with irrigation and aspiration. If the anterior chamber shallows, multiple 10-0 nylon sutures should be placed to ensure a watertight wound. Inferiorly located cortex should be removed first as the risk of capsular injury is greatest with removal of the subincisional material near the 12:00 meridian (Fig. 11.25). To facilitate superior cortical cleanup, a U-shaped cannula may be helpful. Removal of residual 12:00 cortex may be postponed until after IOL implantation, which frequently loosens the attachment to the peripheral posterior capsule.

IOL Implantation

We prefer implantation of a large optic, 6.5- or 7.0-mm polymethyl methacrylate IOL with prolene haptics, particularly in eyes with large pupils that constrict poorly. After filling the capsular bag and anterior chamber with viscoelastic material, the surgeon grasps the IOL optic with a Kelman-McPherson tying forceps (Duckworth & Kent USA Ltd., St. Louis, MO) and introduces the IOL into the anterior chamber. After positioning the inferior haptic within the capsular bag, he rotates the IOL 45 degrees clockwise to further direct the leading haptic into the capsular bag. The posterior haptic that protrudes from the cataract incision is stabilized with a 0.12 mm Castroviejo forceps and grasped with the Kelman-McPherson forceps. The forceps are used to push the superior haptic and IOL into the capsular bag. Either a Sinskey hook or the forceps may be used to rotate the IOL haptics 180 degrees along the 3:00 and 9:00 meridians. An intraocular miotic, such as acetylcholine, is injected to constrict the pupil and prevent IOL capture.

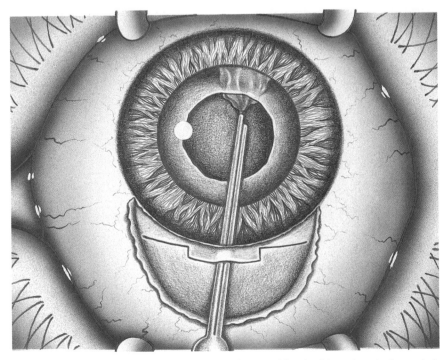

FIGURE 11.25. Extracapsular cataract extraction combined with trabeculectomy. Irrigation and aspiration of residual cortex, automated or manual technique.

Trabeculectomy

Inner block removal with a Vannas scissors or a Descemet's punch and peripheral iridectomy are completed as described previously in Chapter 5 (Fig. 11.26). The anterior chamber should be filled with viscoelastic material during inner block removal to prevent loss of anterior chamber depth.

Wound Closure

Prior to suturing of the trabeculectomy flap and the limbal incision, the remaining viscoelastic material should be removed. The scleral flap is closed with interrupted 10-0 nylon sutures at each corner and the limbal incision with figure-of-8 or multiple 10-0 nylon sutures (Fig. 11.27). The surgeon judges the rate of aqueous outflow by drying the trabeculectomy flap with a cellulose sponge as BSS is injected through the paracentesis. Additional sutures are placed as needed to ensure a formed anterior chamber and moderate aqueous flow. The conjunctiva is closed with a continuous running 10-0 nylon or 8-0 polyglactin 910 (Vicryl, Ethicon Products Worldwide, Somerville, NJ) suture or multiple interrupted 10-0 nylon mattress sutures. The bleb should remain formed and the conjunctival wound watertight after filling of the anterior chamber with BSS.

Postoperative Medications

Subconjunctival corticosteroids and broad-spectrum antibiotics are usually injected in the subconjunctival space. To minimize postoperative inflammation, topical 1% prednisolone acetate should be instilled every 2 hours during waking hours. The surgeon should remind the patient and family members to discontinue all preoperative glaucoma medications.

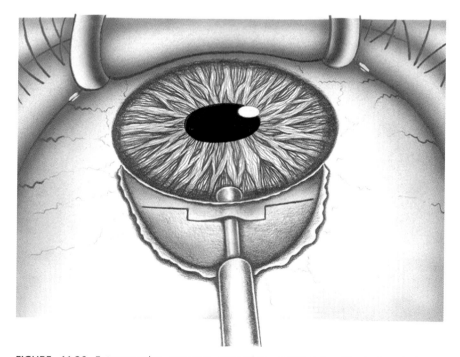

FIGURE 11.26. Extracapsular cataract extraction combined with trabeculectomy. Inner block removal with a Kelly Descemet's punch (Storz Instruments, Bausch & Lomb, Rochester, NY).

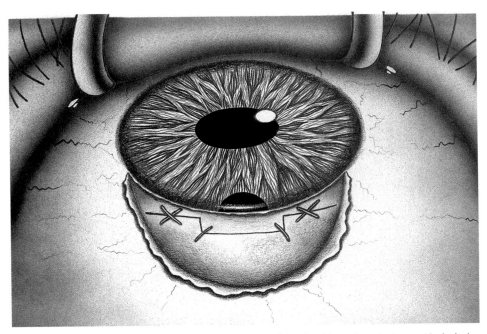

FIGURE 11.27. Extracapsular cataract extraction combined with trabeculectomy. Limbal closure with interrupted 10-0 nylon sutures at corners of trabeculectomy flap and figure-of-8 suture at each side of the flap. Additional sutures are placed as needed to secure the wound.

SURGICAL PEARLS

- Discontinue topical miotics before surgery.
- Evaluate pupillary dilation preoperatively to plan surgery.
- Preoperatively evaluate lid position and orbital anatomy to consider superior tunnel incision versus temporal clear corneal selection.
- Limit the use of topical anesthesia to cooperative patients with adequate pupillary dilation.
- Consider the quicker one-site combined procedure rather than two-site surgery, particularly when beginning combined cataract/glaucoma surgery.
- Limit the use of cautery so as to minimize postoperative inflammation.
- Consider the easier and quicker fornix-based approach instead of the limbus-based combined procedure.
- Consider placing the IOL in the sulcus instead of in the capsular bag in patients with exfoliation syndrome. Weak zonular attachment and late capsular bag dehiscence can result in IOL dislocation.
- Consider the use of antimetabolites in combined cataract/glaucoma surgery (see Chapter 9).

REFERENCES

1. Schuman JS. Surgical management of coexisting cataract and glaucoma. *Ophth Surg Lasers* 1996;27: 45–59.
2. Shields MB. Another reevaluation of combined cataract and glaucoma surgery. *Am J Ophthalmol* 1993;115:806–811.
3. Koch PS. *Mastering phacoemulsification; a simplified manual of strategies for the spring, crack and stop and chop technique,* 4th ed. Thorofare, NJ: Slack, 1994.
4. Casson RJ, Salmon JF. Combined surgery in the treatment of patients with cataract and primary open-angle glaucoma. *J Catar Refract Surg* 2001;27:1854–1863.

12

GLAUCOMA AQUEOUS HUMOR DRAINAGE DEVICES

Although 5-fluorouracil (5-FU) and mitomycin C (MMC) have improved the success of trabeculectomy in patients whose conditions have poor prognoses, glaucoma drainage devices, also known as aqueous tube shunts, are an option for those with extensive limbal scarring and iris neovascularization.

MECHANISM OF ACTION

A medical-grade silicone rubber tube shunts aqueous humor from the anterior chamber to an encapsulated space that forms around an equatorially located plate (1). The fibrous capsule, composed of densely compacted collagen fibers, develops 3 to 5 weeks after implantation. Unlike the typical thin limbal filtering blebs with conjunctival microcysts, the walls of the encapsulated cavity are thicker, more vascular, and less permeable to aqueous humor. The capsular thickness and volume determine the rate of aqueous humor outflow and extent of intraocular pressure (IOP) lowering. Generally, the larger the plate surface area, the lower the IOP. The double-plated Molteno implant (IOP, Inc., Costa Mesa, CA) provides better IOP control than the single-plate device (2). The fact that the 350-mm^2 and 500-mm^2 Baerveldt implants (Pharmacia Ophthalmology, Pharmacia Corporation, Kalamazoo, MI) provide similar IOP control suggests that further reduction is not achieved beyond a certain surface area (3). The 425-mm^2 and 500-mm^2 implants are no longer commercially available.

TYPES OF DRAINAGE DEVICES

Glaucoma drainage devices vary in composition, shape, and surface area; however, all shunt aqueous humor from the anterior chamber to an equatorial cavity. In the immediate postoperative period, before development of resistance in the capsular wall, the rate of aqueous humor outflow must be restricted to prevent postoperative hypotony. A valve (Ahmed Drainage Device, New World Medical, Rancho Cucamonga, CA, or Krupin Valve, Hood Laboratories, Pembroke, MA) or a suture around or within a valveless device (Molteno Device, IOP, Inc., Costa Mesa, CA or Baerveldt Glaucoma Implant, Pharmacia Ophthalmology, Pharmacia Corporation, Kalamazoo, MI) limits aqueous flow. Table 12.1 summarizes the features of commonly used glaucoma drainage devices.

Nonvalved Devices

Molteno Implant

The single-plate adult Molteno implant consists of a circular rigid 135 mm^2 polypropylene plate connected to a valveless flexible silicone rubber tube. Nonabsorbable sutures

TABLE 12.1. SHUNT SPECIFICATIONS

Shunt	Type/Resistance	Tube Materials	Tube Diameter (Outer/Inner)	Plate Material	Plate Surface Area (mm^2)	Plate Shape
Molteno	Nonrestrictive/none	Silicone	0.63/0.30 mm	Polypropylene	135, double plate 270	Round
Krupin	Restrictive/slit valve	Silastic	0.58/0.38 mm	Silicone	180	Oval
					300 (360-degree band)	Rectangular
Baerveldt	Nonrestrictive/none	Silicone	0.63/0.30 mm	Silicone	250, 350, 425[a], 500[a]	Curved
Ahmed	Restrictive/Venturi valve	Silastic	0.63/0.30 mm	Polypropylene/ silicone valve	184, double plate 364	Pear
OptiMed	Restrictive/microtubules	Silicone	0.56/0.30 mm	Silicone/ PMMA matrix	140	Rectangular
ACTEB	Nonrestrictive/none	Silastic	0.64/0.30 mm	Silicone band	300 (360-degree band)	Rectangular
Joseph	Restrictive/slit valve	Silicone	0.64/0.30 mm	Silicone	765 (360-degree band)	Rectangular
White	Restrictive/two valves	Silicone	0.64/0.32 mm	Silicone	280	Round

[a]425 mm^2 and 500 mm^2 are not commercially available.
From *EyeNet* 6(8), September 2002, p. 32, with permission.

passed through positioning holes in the plate secure the device to the globe. A 270-mm^2 Molteno double-plate implant is available in right and left eye models. A bridging silicone tube connects the two single plates; however, only one plate is directly connected to the anterior chamber. The four-plate implant is no longer commercially available. A smaller pediatric implant may be used in smaller than usual eyes, and in eyes after cyclodestructive surgery.

Baerveldt Implant

This flexible elliptically shaped silicone rubber device, available in 250 mm^2 and 350 mm^2 sizes (model BG103-250, BG101-350), can be implanted through a single-quadrant conjunctival incision (4). The original plate design was associated with the frequent development of large encapsulated blebs and noncommitant motility problems (5). The current version with holes in the plate has resulted in a lower bleb profile and reduced incidence of postoperative diplopia. A specially modified Baerveldt implant has been developed for implantation through the *pars plana* (BG102-350) (Chapter 13).

Valved Devices

Krupin Valve

A silicone tube slit valve maintains the immediate postoperative IOP between 9 and 11 mm Hg, according to the manufacturer, without the use of a suture to limit aqueous outflow. The tube is connected to an oval plate with an area of 183 mm^2.

Ahmed Valve

The Ahmed valve consists of a silicone tube attached to either a single 184-mm^2 polypropylene plate a 364-mm^2 two plate version designed to maintain an IOP between 8 and 14 mm Hg (6). A Venturi style valve limits the rate of aqueous humor outflow.

INDICATIONS

Glaucoma drainage devices are usually used in eyes whose conditions have poor prognoses for trabeculectomy, such as after failed filtering surgery, neovascular glaucoma, inflammatory glaucoma, glaucoma associated with aphakia or pseudophakia, after vitreoretinal surgery glaucoma, and after penetrating keratoplasty.

SURGICAL TECHNIQUE

The surgical approach to implantation is similar with most glaucoma drainage devices. The device selection will dictate incision size and whether the tube must be occluded.

Surgical Exposure

A clear cornea traction suture placed anteriorly to the anticipated site of tube entry permits rotation of the globe to provide adequate visualization (Chapter 5). Alternatively, a suture may be passed through the perilimbal sclera if a penetrating keratoplasty was recently performed.

Conjunctival Incision

A single-quadrant incision, usually three or four clock hours wide, is usually sufficient for single-plate Molteno implant, Baerveldt implant, single-plate Ahmed valve, or Krupin disc valve implantation. The double-plate Molteno implant and double-plate Ahmed valve require a larger incision (180 degrees). We prefer a fornix-based conjunctival and Tenon's capsule flap. With extensive limbal scarring, a sharp blade may be used to dissect the conjunctiva that is usually recessed from the normal attachment. The surgeon bluntly dissects Tenon's capsule from underlying sclera posteriorly to the rectus muscle insertions with round-tipped West-cott scissors (Storz Instruments, Bausch & Lomb, Rochester, NY) (Fig. 12.1).

Priming of the Implant

The surgeon tests the drainage device patency and valve function by injecting balanced salt solution (BSS, Alcon Laboratories, Fort Worth, TX) through a 30-gauge cannula until flow is observed. This maneuver is particularly important to test the function of implants with valves.

Positioning the Plate

Implantation of single-plate devices is usually easiest in the superotemporal quadrant. With double-plate devices, the scleral surface in the superior nasal and superior temporal quadrants must be prepared. The anterior border of the plate should be sutured to the sclera with

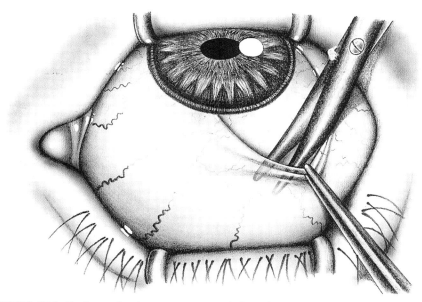

FIGURE 12.1. Drainage implant surgery. Fornix-based conjunctival flap and Tenon's capsule peritomy with nontoothed forceps and Westcott scissors (Storz Instruments, Bausch & Lomb, Rochester, NY).

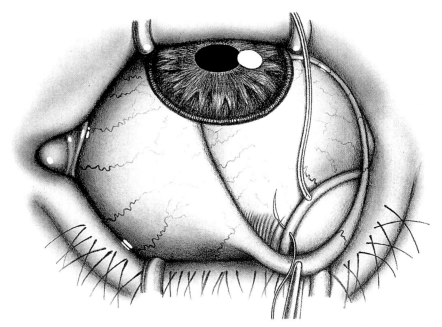

FIGURE 12.2. Drainage implant surgery. Attachment of the plate to the sclera with two interrupted 9-0 nylon sutures through anterior positioning holes. Knots should be buried to minimize conjunctival erosion.

9-0 nylon sutures on a spatula needle, approximately 8 to 9 mm posterior to the surgical limbus (Fig. 12.2).

Scleral Flap Dissection

If donor material, such as glycerin-preserved cornea or sclera, is unavailable, a split thickness, that is, a 4 × 5 mm scleral flap, may be prepared to cover the tube (Fig. 12.3). Dis-

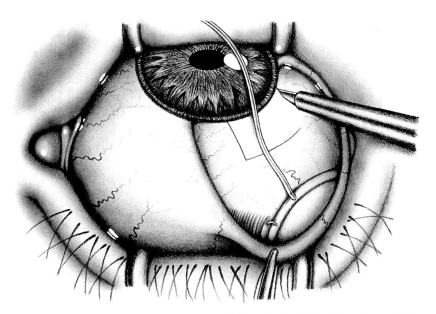

FIGURE 12.3. Drainage implant surgery. Outlining of scleral flap dissection to 80% depth with sharp blade.

section of a scleral flap may be difficult in eyes after previous filtering surgery. If the scleral flap is not sufficiently thick, the tube may erode through it and the overlying conjunctiva. We strongly recommend using preserved donor cornea, sclera, dura, or pericardium (Tranzgraft, New World Medical, Rancho Cucamonga, CA) to cover the tube (7).

PREVENTION OF IMMEDIATE POSTOPERATIVE HYPOTONY

Unless aqueous humor outflow is restricted in devices without valves, complications may develop as a result of marked early postoperative hypotony. To minimize this problem, the device may be temporarily occluded or implanted in two stages.

Two-Stage Procedure

In the first stage, as originally described by Molteno, the plate is fixed to the sclera and the tube is temporarily sutured to the sclera or tucked beneath one of the rectus muscles without entering the anterior chamber. After a thick-walled capsule has formed around the drainage plate in 4 to 6 weeks that will minimize hypotony, the tube is inserted into the anterior chamber and covered with a patch graft in the second stage. This technique has been demonstrated to minimize postoperative hypotony and choroidal effusion in eyes of children with Sturge-Weber syndrome (8). After completing the second stage, the surgeon injects a viscoelastic material into the anterior chamber to minimize hypotony in these eyes that are prone to develop large choroidal effusions. To control the IOP before tube insertion, either preoperative medications must be continued or a temporary drainage site (orphan trabeculectomy) must be made in an adjacent quadrant (Fig. 12.4).

One-Stage Procedure

Two techniques are used to limit aqueous humor outflow when nonvalved devices are inserted in a single stage. Some surgeons may further limit outflow with valved devices by

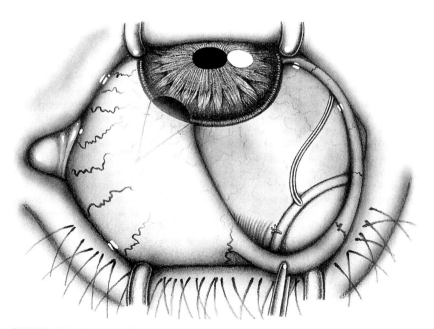

FIGURE 12.4. Drainage implant surgery: two-stage procedure. Attachment of plate to sclera and positioning of tube under lateral rectus muscle insertion. Trabeculectomy without intraoperative antimetabolites may be placed for temporary intraocular pressure control (orphan trabeculectomy).

temporarily closing the tube with a suture. This may be performed if early postoperative hypotony poses a special risk for suprachoroidal hemorrhage, such as in eyes with very high preoperative pressures.

Tube Ligation in the Sub-Tenon's Space

We ligate the tube with an absorbable suture, such as 5-0 or 7-0 polyglactin (Vicryl, Ethicon Products Worldwide, Johnson & Johnson, Somerville, NJ), placed between the posterior edge of the scleral patch and the anterior border of the plate (Fig. 12.5). Before implantation, the surgeon checks the tube for watertight occlusion by injecting BSS into the lumen through the 30-gauge cannula after the first triple-knot throw of a surgeon's knot. The final two throws in the knot are completed after demonstration that BSS cannot be forced through the tube. Care should be taken to avoid cutting the tube when tightening the suture. Heavy nonserrated straight locking needle holders (Product Number 3850, 3852, or 3861, Storz Instruments, Bausch & Lomb, Rochester, NY) facilitate grasping the suture ends and tying. The suture usually absorbs by the 35th through 42nd postoperative day after a fibrous capsule has formed around the plate.

Tube Ligation in the Anterior Chamber

A polypropylene or nylon suture may be tied around the tube near the tip before the tube is introduced into the anterior chamber. The surgeon applies low-power, short-duration, large-spot argon laser burns to the intraocular portion of the suture to loosen it and initiate outflow after the capsule has formed.

As with the two-stage technique, the IOP must be controlled with preoperative medications until the tube is patent. Alternatively, a temporary filtering site in an adjacent quadrant (orphan trabeculectomy) or multiple tube slits between the suture and the tube tip permit aqueous outflow to lower immediate postoperative IOP. Two or three through-and-through (double-wall) perforations are made in the center of the tube with a spatula needle.

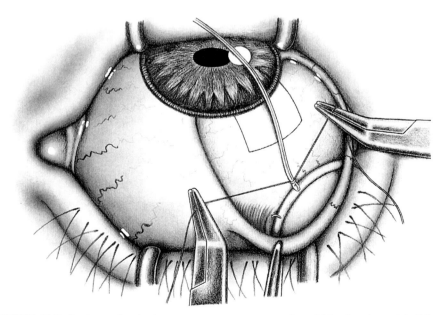

FIGURE 12.5. Drainage implant surgery: one-stage procedure. Tube ligation with 7-0 absorbable suture for watertight closure.

Tube Insertion into the Anterior Chamber

The surgeon places the tube in its unbent or natural position over the peripheral cornea and cuts it with scissors to produce an upward-facing bevel (Fig. 12.6). The tube tip, equidistant from the limbus and the pupillary border, should extend approximately 2.0 to 3.0 mm into the anterior chamber. If the tube is longer than desired, it should be removed and trimmed. If the tube is not sufficiently long, a tube extender (New World Medical, Rancho Cucamonga, CA) or a 20-gauge angiocatheter (Becton–Dickinson, Franklin Lakes, NJ) may be used for lengthening. The surgeon makes a paracentesis parallel to the iris plane for the tube insertion with a sharp 23-gauge needle, connected to a syringe with viscoelastic material or BSS (Fig. 12.7). A small amount of viscoelastic material injected into the anterior chamber through the paracentesis tract may facilitate tube insertion. The chamber should not be overfilled since the increased depth may not accurately reflect the position of the tube postoperatively. With two nontoothed forceps, the surgeon inserts the tube through the paracentesis into the anterior chamber. Alternatively, specially designed forceps, such as the tubing introducer forceps (Assi, Westbury, NY), may be used. In an aphakic and vitrectomized eye, the tube may be inserted through the pars plana (see Chapter 13).

Suturing of the Tube

Some surgeons prefer suturing the tube to the sclera with one or two 9-0 or 10-0 nylon sutures (Fig. 12.8). These sutures fix the tube and do not close it. With a scleral flap, one interrupted suture is placed at each corner and the knots are buried (Fig. 12.9). When donor tissue is used, a 4 × 5 mm patch graft, centered over the tube, is fixed to the sclera with either 10-0 nylon or 7-0 polyglactin 910 sutures at each corner (Fig. 12.10). As with the scleral flap, all knots should be buried to avoid damaging the conjunctiva.

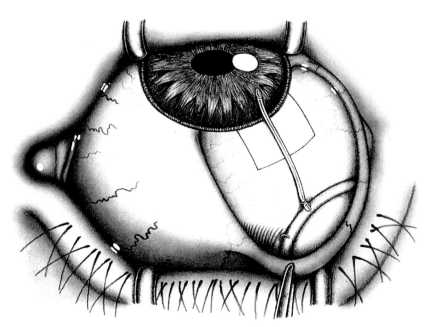

FIGURE 12.6. Drainage implant surgery. Beveled tube tip after trimming. The bevel should face the cornea (anteriorly) and extend approximately 2.0 to 3.0 mm into the anterior chamber.

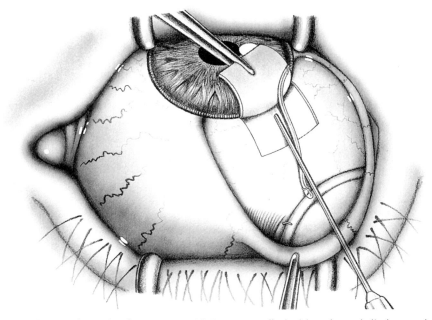

FIGURE 12.7. Drainage implant surgery. 23-Gauge needle incision through limbus under scleral flap, parallel to the iris plane for tube insertion. Viscoelastic material may be injected to maintain anterior chamber depth.

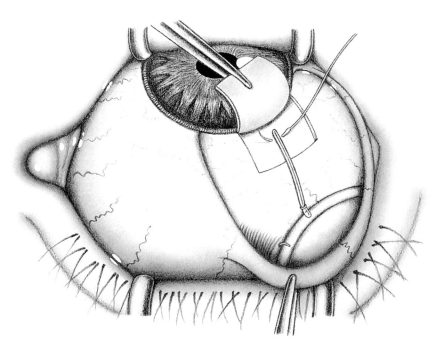

FIGURE 12.8. Drainage implant surgery. Tube attachment to the sclera with interrupted 9-0 nylon sutures.

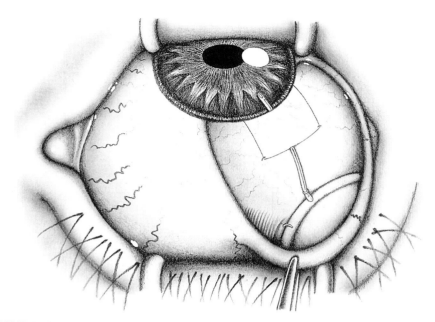

FIGURE 12.9. Drainage implant surgery. Scleral flap closure over tube with interrupted absorbable sutures and buried knots.

Conjunctival Closure

With the fornix-based flap, Tenon's capsule and conjunctiva are closed with either horizontal interrupted mattress, figure-of-8, or continuous sutures (Fig. 12.11). Conjunctival closure may be assessed by injecting BSS through the paracentesis tract and inspecting the wound with a cellulose sponge as described in Chapter 5 (see Fig. 5.39).

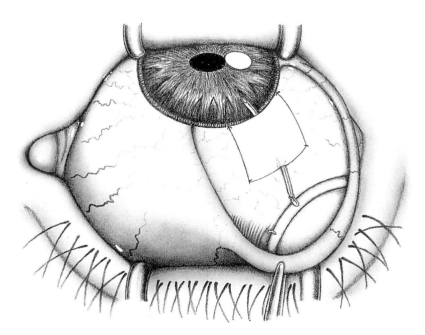

FIGURE 12.10. Drainage implant surgery. Donor patch graft material: sclera, cornea, dura mater, or pericardium to cover the tube. Knots at the four corners should be buried to minimize damaging the overlying conjunctiva.

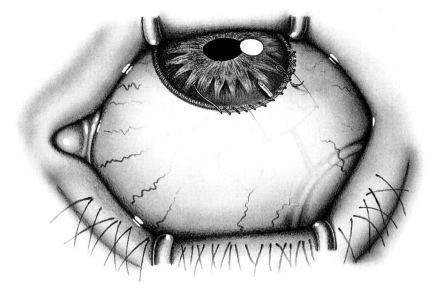

FIGURE 12.11. Drainage implant surgery. Continuous absorbable suture closure of Tenon's capsule and the conjunctiva.

Postoperative Subconjunctival Injections

An antibiotic, such as gentamicin sulfate (20 mg), and a corticosteroid, such as dexamethasone sodium phosphate (2 mg), are usually given, although many surgeons prefer a combination corticosteroid–antibiotic ointment.

POSTOPERATIVE CARE

Postoperative care is similar to that given after trabeculectomy. Topical 1% prednisolone acetate, 4 to 6 times daily, during the first 2 to 3 weeks is slowly tapered over the next 4 to 5 weeks. A topical broad-spectrum antibiotic, such as polymyxin–trimethoprim, is usually applied until the conjunctival incision is healed. Cycloplegics are not routinely used. If a ligature is used to restrict aqueous outflow through the tube, preoperative glaucoma medications are continued until the suture absorbs.

COMPLICATIONS

Although complications of hyphema, choroidal detachment, choroidal hemorrhage, or malignant glaucoma may occur after any glaucoma filtering procedure (Chapters 7, 8, and 10), glaucoma drainage devices are associated with a special group of intraoperative and postoperative problems.

Intraoperative Complications of Glaucoma Drainage Devices

Inadvertent Tube Cutting

Excessive force applied during suture tightening may bisect the tube. If this happens the entire implant may be replaced or the surgeon may repair the cut with a tube extender or a 22-gauge angiocatheter (9). The portion of the tube that will enter the anterior chamber and the posterior portion attached to the plate both fit into the tube extender or angiocatheter. If the anterior portion of the tube cannot be used, then a piece of trimmed pediatric lacrimal tubing (internal diameter 0.3 mm, external diameter 0.64 mm; Dow Corning, Midland, MI) may be used to lengthen the tube.

Improper Introduction of the Tube

The tube may touch the cornea, iris, or lens if introduced at the improper angle. In this case, the tube should be removed and the original entry site closed if aqueous leakage is noted. A new entry parallel to the iris plane should be made with a 23-gauge needle.

Leakage Around the Tube

If the limbal paracentesis is substantially wider than the tube, then aqueous humor may flow around the sides of the tube and result in postoperative hypotony. If excessive leakage cannot be reduced with interrupted sutures around the tube, the tube should be removed, the entry site closed, and another paracentesis tract made.

Postoperative Complications of the Glaucoma Drainage Devices

Hypotony

Aqueous humor leakage around the tube at the point of limbal insertion, a loosely tied occluding suture, and an improperly functioning valve may explain excessively low IOP immediately after surgery (10). Earlier than usual absorption of the ligature suture may also lead to low IOP if a thick capsule has not formed around the plate. Hypotony may result in a shallow anterior chamber and cornea–tube contact. It is necessary to reform the anterior chamber with viscoelastic material and drain choroidal detachments if present.

Obstruction of the Tube

Iris, vitreous, blood, or fibrin may obstruct the tube in the immediate postoperative period (11). If vitreous is present within the tube, neodymium:yttrium-argon-garnet (Nd:YAG) vitreolysis will not relieve the blockage and an anterior vitrectomy should be performed (Fig. 12.12). The tube tip should be irrigated with sterile BSS introduced through a 30-gauge cannula to demonstrate patency.

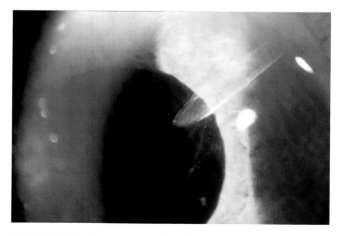

FIGURE 12.12. Blockage of tube with strands of vitreous after spontaneous tube suturelysis associated with immediate hypotony and acute intraocular pressure elevation. (Reprinted from Parrish RK II, ed. *University of Miami Bascom Palmer Eye Institute Atlas of Ophthalmology.* Philadelphia: Current Medicine, 2000:231, with permission.)

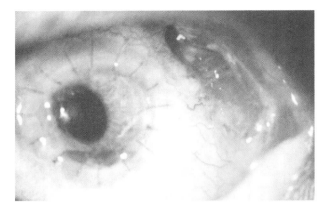

FIGURE 12.13. Postoperative extrusion of Molteno drainage device (IOP, Inc., Costa Mesa, CA) associated with large conjunctival dehiscence in an eye after multiple procedures involving the conjunctiva.

Tube or Plate Extrusion

The tube or the plate may erode through the conjunctiva, particularly if a relaxing incision was made at the lateral extent of the fornix-based incision and exposure may be a risk factor for late-onset endophthalmitis (12). Late extrusion usually leads to removal of the drainage device, although an attempt may be made to place a patch graft over the area of exposure before closing the conjunctiva (Fig. 12.13). Tube erosion, a more common problem, occurs if a thin scleral flap was dissected or if the patch graft absorbs. Surgical repair with a new patch graft should be used to cover the tube, and Tenon's capsule should be closed before suturing the conjunctiva over the graft. Closure of the conjunctiva alone is inadequate and will result in recurrent erosion. If erosion recurs, it may be necessary to use a different quadrant for the tube's entry or to remove the device.

INTRAOCULAR PRESSURE ELEVATION

Early postoperative IOP elevation may be explained by valve failure, which occurs if the device was not primed before implantation. If the IOP remains elevated after 6 weeks and the area over the plate is flat, the surgeon should inspect the tube tip for obstruction. If no obstruction is identified, the conjunctiva should be opened and the valve inspected. If

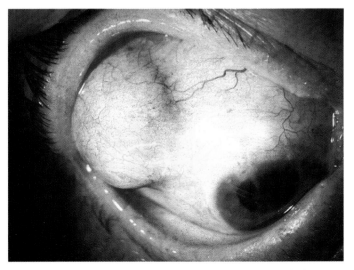

FIGURE 12.14. Encapsulation of bleb around Ahmed drainage implant (New World Medical, Ranch Cucamonga, CA) 1 year after surgery. Note high profile and limited bleb extension.

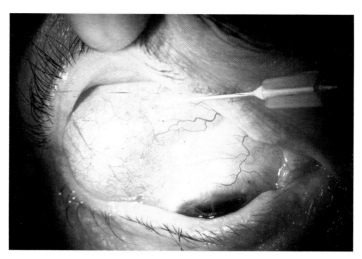

FIGURE 12.15. Needling of encapsulated bleb with immediate enlargement of bleb after perforation of bleb wall. (Same eye as in Fig. 12.14.)

iris obstructs the tip, repositioning is necessary. Anterior vitrectomy should be performed for incarceration of vitreous. A transient hypertensive phase occurs in the absence of tube occlusion and is likely explained by remodeling of the scar tissue around the plate. Hypotensive drugs should be used during this period to control IOP. If an extremely thick capsule forms around the plate, removal of a portion of the capsule wall or needling may be performed as described in Chapters 8 and 10 however, these procedures do not usually result in permanent IOP reduction (Figs. 12.14 and 12.15). We prefer the implantation of a second drainage device, usually in the inferonasal quadrant (13).

LATE POSTOPERATIVE TUBE MIGRATION

The tube tip may come into contact with the iris or cornea. Mechanical injury to the corneal endothelium may result from eye blinking and rubbing. If this occurs the tube should be repositioned or trimmed (Figs. 12.16 and 12.17).

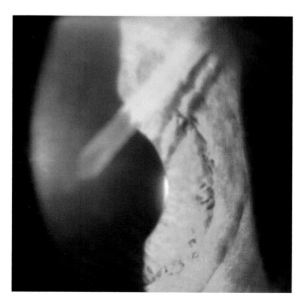

FIGURE 12.16. Corneal endothelial contact with tube tip and overlying corneal stromal edema.

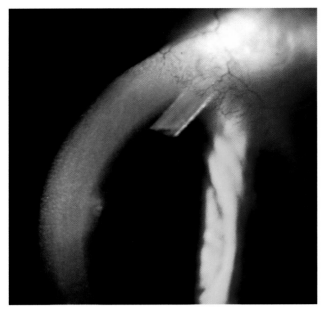

FIGURE 12.17. Appearance after trimming tube tip with resolution of corneal edema.

SURGICAL PEARLS

- Widely expose the scleral surface and remove adhesions of the intramuscular septum from the rectus muscle insertions.
- Remember that the superior, lateral, inferior, and medial rectus muscles are approximately 10 mm wide at their insertions.
- Remember the location of the rectus muscles insertions at the spiral of Tillaux: medial 5.5 mm, inferior 6.5 mm, lateral 6.7 mm, superior 7.2 to 7.7 mm. This is particularly important after previous retinal detachment surgery.
- Test the patency of the implant and valve function before implantation.
- Confirm the watertight nature of the temporary occluding suture around the tube before permanently tying it off.
- Pass the needle and suture through the sclera first and then through the fixation hole of the implant.
- Avoid dissecting a scleral flap to cover the tube. The pressure of the tube against the flap may cause progressive thinning and late conjunctival perforation.
- Use glycerin-preserved cornea, sclera, or specially prepared cadaveric pericardium or dura mater (Tutorplast, New World Medical, Rancho Cucamonga, CA).
- Use a 23-gauge sharp needle to make the paracentesis tract parallel to the iris for the tube implantation. Bend the needle shaft so that you can hold it comfortably like a pencil.
- Slightly enlarge the posterior end of the tract with the 23-gauge needle tip to make insertion easier. If the anterior chamber shallows, reform it before attempting reinsertion of the tube.
- Inject viscoelastic material in the paracentesis tract to facilitate tube insertion.

GLAUCOMA SURGERY AFTER PENETRATING KERATOPLASTY

Elevated IOP frequently complicates the postoperative course of penetrating keratoplasty and may contribute to graft failure. The pressure lowering strategy depends on the mechanism of elevation. Filtering surgery is indicated when medical treatment fails to control IOP. As standard trabeculectomy alone usually fails to reduce IOP, intraoperative 5-FU or MMC are frequently used. If postoperative 5-FU injections are given, the corneal and conjunctival epithelium must be very carefully monitored for signs of toxicity. Tube shunt surgery may be performed instead of trabeculectomy (6). If the tube is placed in the anterior chamber, its orientation should be parallel to the iris with the tip directed away from the corneal endothelium. In an aphakic or pseudophakic eye, the tube may be inserted through the *pars plana* after pars plana vitrectomy. Cyclodestructive procedures usually lower IOP, but may induce intraocular inflammation, cystoid macular edema or graft failure. We reserve cyclodestruction for the treatment of eyes with poor visual acuity after failed tube shunt surgery.

REFERENCES

1. Walsh JB, Muldoon TO: Glaucoma associated with retinal and vitreoretinal disorders. In: Ritch R, Shields MB, Krupin T, eds. *The glaucomas*, 2nd ed. St. Louis: Mosby, 1996:1055–1071.
2. Ando F. Intraocular hypertension resulting from pupillary block by silicone oil. *Am J Ophthalmol* 1985;99:87–88.
3. Nazemi PP, Chong LP, Varma R, et al. Migration of intraocular silicone oil into the subconjunctival space and orbit through an Ahmed glaucoma valve. *Am J Ophthalmol* 2001;132:929–931.
4. Scott IU, Alexandrakis G, Flynn HW Jr, et al. Combined pars plana vitrectomy and glaucoma drainage implant placement for refractory glaucoma. *Am J Ophthalmol* 2000;129:334–341.
5. Tomey KF, Traverso CE. The glaucomas in aphakia and pseudophakia. *Surv Ophthalmol* 1991;36:79–112.
6. Sherwood MB, Smith MF, Driebe WT Jr, et al. Drainage tube implants in the treatment of glaucoma following penetrating keratoplasty. *Ophth Surg* 1993;24:185–189.

LASER PERIPHERAL IRIDOTOMY, LASER TRABECULOPLASTY, AND LASER IRIDOPLASTY

LASER PERIPHERAL IRIDOTOMY

Introduction: Indications

Laser peripheral iridotomy has largely replaced surgical iridectomy because it has fewer risks and may be performed in the office under topical anesthesia. Indications include acute angle-closure glaucoma, the fellow eye in a patient with acute angle closure, and chronic angle-closure glaucoma with pupillary block. Iridotomy may be performed to determine if an angle closure is due to pupillary block in eyes with nanophthalmos, suspected plateau iris configuration, iris pigment epithelial cysts, anterior subluxation of the crystalline lens, pseudoexfoliation, after scleral buckling surgery for retinal detachment, central retinal vein occlusion, and panretinal photocoagulation. Iridotomy may deepen the anterior chamber in eyes with narrow angles and improve the view of the surgeon for argon laser trabeculoplasty. Angle closure without pupillary block, such as iridocorneal endothelium (ICE) syndrome, neovascular glaucoma, epithelialization of the anterior chamber, and sulfonamide (topiramate, Topomax)–related ciliary body edema, should not be managed with iridotomy.

Technique

Topical 2% pilocarpine hydrochloride should be instilled before iridotomy if choroidal effusion or ciliary body swelling is not suspected. Miosis stretches the iris and facilitates peripheral treatment. α_2-Adrenergic agonists, such as apraclonidine (Iopidine, Alcon, Fort Worth, TX) or brimonidine (Alphagan, Allergan, Irvine, CA), instilled 1 hour before and immediately after the procedure minimize IOP elevation. These medications may reduce iris bleeding during neodymium:yttrium-argon-garnet (Nd:YAG) laser iridotomy. The procedure, performed under topical anesthesia, can be performed with either argon or Nd:YAG laser (1). An iridotomy contact lens, such as the planoconvex bifocal Abraham lens (Ocular Instruments, Bellevue, WA), decreases the spot size, increases the power density, and magnifies the iris. The lens also stabilizes the eye and maintains the palpebral aperture during treatment.

Location

With the patient comfortably seated, the surgeon selects an iris crypt or atrophic area in the nasal or superior quadrant. When placed near the 12:00 location, the eyelid covers the iridotomy and minimizes the likelihood of stray light or "ghost images." Temporal iridotomies should be avoided to prevent an inadvertent macular injury. Iridotomies should be placed as peripherally as possible, but just anterior to arcus senilis that may obscure visualization. Because bubbles may form with argon treatment and interfere with focusing of the laser beam, we prefer treating slightly nasal to the 12 o'clock position (Fig. 14.1).

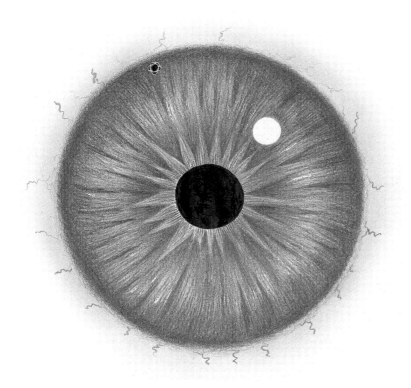

FIGURE 14.1. Laser peripheral iridotomy—left eye. Location in the superior and nasal peripheral iris at 11:00 position.

Laser Type

The laser power settings, spot size, and duration are dependent on the energy source, delivery system, and iris characteristics. With an argon laser, a 50-μm spot, power setting between 500 and 1200 mW, and duration of 0.02 to 0.2 second are usually sufficient to perforate the iris. Brown irides that intensely absorb the argon laser wavelength are usually easier to perforate than blue irides. Initial argon treatment of lightly pigmented irides with a few longer duration spots (0.3 to 0.4 second) and higher power (1200 to 1500 mW) heats the iris pigment epithelium and thins the overlying stroma. After completing this maneuver, the usual argon parameters are chosen to complete the iridotomy. Alternatively, the Nd:YAG laser may be used in lightly pigmented eyes.

With either laser, maintenance of sharp focus on the iris surface is necessary to efficiently complete the treatment. If the surgeon does not focus the laser beam through the center of the bifocal segment in the contact lens, an elliptical spot will be produced with a diminished power density in comparison with that in a perfectly circular spot. Frequently, aqueous humor passes from the posterior to the anterior chamber through the opening and pushes the iris pigment epithelium in a "pigmentary cascade." The anterior lens capsule or the zonules should be observed through the iridotomy and a red reflex seen with retroillumination through the pupil. After the initial perforation, the pigment epithelial remnants at the iridotomy base are removed.

Treatment with the Nd:YAG laser is less dependent on iris color. The peripheral treatment location is identical to that with the argon laser to avoid damage to the anterior lens capsule. The risk of retinal damage is reduced by correctly focusing through the contact lens, and by focusing the beam away from the macula, particularly when the iris has been perforated. Usually 1 to 10 shots with a power setting of 2 to 5 mJ delivered through a contact Abraham Nd:YAG lens coated for the Nd:YAG wavelength (Ocular Instruments, Bellevue, WA) is effective. Mild iris bleeding is stopped by the application of compression with the contact lens.

Postoperative Management

After iridotomy, apraclonidine or brimonidine is instilled to minimize the likelihood of an intraocular pressure (IOP) spike. The IOP should be checked 1 to 2 hours after treatment. Prednisolone acetate 1% is applied 4 times daily for a week to reduce postoperative inflammation. After the iridotomy gonioscopy should be repeated to reassess the angle.

Complications

Complications, usually of a mild nature, infrequently occur with argon or Nd:YAG laser iridotomy. Mild anterior segment inflammation is generally temporary and usually controlled with topical anti-inflammatory agents. The Nd:YAG laser may produce self-limited iris bleeding more commonly than the argon. A transient corneal opacity may be produced by a misfocused shot or by a very shallow anterior chamber. In eyes with secondary angle closure and chronic inflammation, posterior synechiae may develop.

ARGON LASER TRABECULOPLASTY

Introduction: Indications

Argon laser trabeculoplasty (ALT) is indicated for the management of uncontrolled open-angle glaucoma, pigmentary glaucoma, and glaucoma associated with exfoliation syndrome. It has also been proposed as initial therapy for primary open-angle glaucoma instead of medical treatment (2) and for intolerant or noncompliant patients. The IOP lowering effect may diminish after 5 years, and the success rate at 10 years is approximately 10%. ALT is not effective in patients with juvenile glaucoma, uveitic glaucoma, traumatic glaucoma, or postsurgical glaucoma.

Surgical Technique

Preoperative 0.5% apraclonidine or 0.2% brimonidine is instilled to minimize an IOP spike. Topical 0.5% proparacaine is usually sufficient, although retrobulbar or peribulbar block may occasionally be required in patients with nystagmus. A gonioscopy lens or a specially designed lens, such as the Ritch trabeculoplasty laser lens (Ocular Instruments, Bellevue, WA) filled with hydroxypropyl methylcellulose 2% as coupling solution precisely focuses the energy. The patient is asked to look toward the mirror of the lens to better expose the angle. The surgeon should be familiar with the angle structures before beginning treatment. Usually 180 degrees of the angle is initially treated. We generally begin with the inferior angle, which is the widest and most pigmented area. We suggest that each surgeon develop a routine to be followed for initial and subsequent treatments. The surgeon should remember the direction of treatment (clockwise or counterclockwise) to reduce the chances of overtreatment. The burns should be placed in the middle of the trabecular meshwork located in the junction between the nonpigmented and the pigmented portions (Fig. 14.2). Forty to fifty applications are delivered to the 180 degrees or half the angle. A spot size of 50 μm and a duration of 0.1 second are selected. The power settings are usually between 400 and 1200 mW. The goal, that is, production of small bubbles or a minimal pigment blanching of the meshwork with the lowest power, may require adjustment of power throughout the procedure. Excessive power settings or posteriorly positioned burns may cause posterior synechiae formation. To avoid this complication, the laser beam should be correctly focused perpendicular to the meshwork. The surgeon may tilt the lens slightly or ask the patient to look toward the mirror in use to assure proper focusing and spot placement.

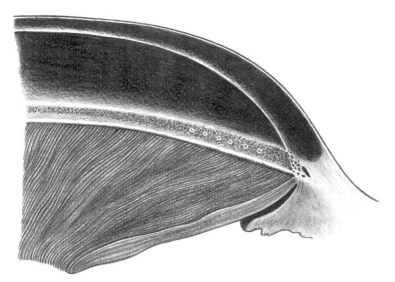

FIGURE 14.2. Argon laser trabeculoplasty. Laser burns at the junction of the anterior (nonpigmented) and posterior (pigmented) trabecular meshwork.

Postoperative Care

Immediately after ALT, apraclonidine or brimonidine is administered to reduce the likelihood of an acute IOP elevation and the IOP is measured in 1 to 2 hours. Topical prednisolone acetate 1% is given 3 to 4 times daily for 5 to 7 days to suppress inflammation. As the IOP lowering effect of argon laser trabeculoplasty may not be apparent for 6 weeks, patients should continue their preoperative antiglaucoma medications postoperatively.

Complications

Complications after argon laser trabeculoplasty are uncommon. An early postoperative IOP spike should be monitored for, particularly in patients with advanced visual field and optic nerve damage. Oral carbonic anhydrase inhibitors or osmotic agents may be required for the management of severe IOP elevation. Mild and transient anterior chamber inflammation is usually controlled with a short course of topical corticosteroids. Posterior synechiae may complicate ALT, particularly in eyes with narrow chamber angles and posteriorly located laser burns. Failure to lower IOP satisfactorily after 180 degrees ALT is an indication for treatment of the remaining angle. Usually the IOP lowering effect cannot be judged until 6 weeks after the first treatment session. The surgeon should remember that the likelihood of success is less with retreatment than initial ALT.

LASER IRIDOPLASTY

The argon laser may be used to alter the configuration of either the central or peripheral iris (3).

Central Iridoplasty: Pupilloplasty and Photomydriasis

Pupilloplasty is used to break an angle closure attack associated with pupillary block when an iridotomy cannot be performed for technical reasons, such as peripheral iris and corneal contact. This treatment distorts the pupillary shape and allows aqueous humor to pass from the posterior to the anterior chamber. Peripheral iridotomy should be performed after the attack has been broken with pupilloplasty and the anterior chamber has deepened. The surgeon places laser applications (200 to 400 μm spot size, 0.2 second duration, with a power of 200 to 300 mW) near the collarette in one quadrant to shrink the iris and alter the pupil.

Photomydriasis is achieved by placing circumferential burns around the pupil to shrink the iris and clear the optical axis in eyes receiving long-term miotic therapy. One or two concentric rings of argon laser spots are applied with a 100 to 150 μm spot size, 0.3 to 0.5 second duration, at a power of 200 to 300 mW.

Peripheral Iridoplasty

Also known as gonioplasty, this procedure flattens the peripheral iris configuration to widen the angle approach.

Indications for Peripheral Iridoplasty

This technique improves angle visualization when a prominent peripheral iris roll prevents having a clear view of the trabecular meshwork for ALT. It may also be used to deepen a narrow peripheral anterior chamber before argon laser iridotomy to minimize thermal corneal endothelial injury. Peripheral iridoplasty is indicated for the treatment of plateau iris syndrome, in which the angle is appositionally closed or occludable after patent iridectomy. Persistent angle closure after iridotomy and associated with choroidal effusion and ciliary body swelling, seen in such conditions as central retinal vein occlusion without neovascularization, nanophthalmos, scleral buckling procedures, or panretinal photocoagulation, may open after peripheral iridoplasty.

Technique

The procedure may be performed with or without a contact lens (the round gonioscopic mirror of a Goldmann style three-mirror contact lens). The laser beam should be directed to the far peripheral iris with a 200-μm spot size, 0.2- to 0.5-second duration, at a 200- to 600-mW power setting. Generally, four to six applications per quadrant are applied to the areas of peripheral anterior synechiae.

SURGICAL PEARLS

Table 14.1 summarizes the usual laser parameters for each procedure. Suturelysis and the Nd:YAG laser disruption of the anterior hyaloid face are also described in this table, as well as in Chapter 8.

- Always perform gonioscopy before selecting the type and location of laser treatment.
- Instill an α_2 agonist agent before and after treatment to minimize an acute IOP spike.
- Make sure that both you and the patient are comfortably seated before beginning treatment. An armrest can be used to support the surgeon's elbow and stabilize the laser delivery.
- Always direct the aiming beam perpendicular to the area being treated.
- Adjust laser parameters based on observed treatment effect. If no result is obtained with the initial settings, recheck the focus and increase the power or duration. If a satisfactory burn cannot be generated, select a new location.
- Consider using both an argon and a Nd:YAG laser to perform iridotomy. Initial low-power argon burns (500 mW) thin the iris stroma and the high-power Nd:YAG laser easily perforates the remaining iris with one or two shots. Pretreatment with the argon laser diminishes iris bleeding associated with the Nd:YAG laser.
- Anticipate more severe than usual inflammation after iridotomy for acute angle closure in deeply pigmented eyes with thick irides. Consider the use of the Nd:YAG laser for iridotomy in these eyes that are prone to angle closure.

Oral analgesia, frequently codeine, is given as needed. Topical 1% atropine sulfate and 1% prednisolone acetate are given for 2 to 4 weeks. Antiglaucoma medication to reduce aqueous humor production is continued until the effect of the cyclodestructive procedure is assessed, usually within 4 weeks. Miotics and topical prostaglandin derivatives should be discontinued postoperatively.

COMPLICATIONS

Complications of cyclodestructive procedures include prolonged intraocular inflammation, permanently reduced central acuity, cataract, macular edema, corneal edema, choroidal detachment, vitreous hemorrhage, focal scleral thinning, and sympathetic ophthalmia. Moderate ocular pain and anterior uveitis in the immediate postoperative period usually responds to the administration of hourly topical 1% prednisolone acetate and twice daily 1% atropine sulfate. The complication of irreversible hypotony is associated with extensive treatment and chronic intraocular inflammation. A conservative approach of applying fewer than the usual number of treatment spots should be followed in eyes with poor prognoses. Because of the possible serious complications, cyclodestructive procedures should be performed with extreme caution in eyes with good visual potential.

SURGICAL PEARLS

- Frankly discuss the potential complications of these procedures with the patient.
- Reserve cyclodestructive procedures for eyes with poor visual acuity potential.
- Consider peribulbar rather than retrobulbar anesthesia.
- Test the cryoprobe and delivery system before beginning treatment.
- Avoid contact between the cryoprobe and the eyelids.
- Remember that the iceball size increases during the 60-second application.
- Do not remove the cryoprobe until the iceball thaws. Premature removal may tear the conjunctiva.
- The G-probe edge should be positioned at the site of the last treatment spot to evenly space the applications.

REFERENCES

1. Prost M. Cyclocryotherapy for glaucoma. Evaluation of techniques. *Surv Ophthalmol* 1983;28: 93–100.
2. Liu GJ, Mizukawa A, Okisaka S. Mechanism of intraocular pressure decrease after contact transscleral continuous-wave Nd:YAG laser cyclophotocoagulation. *Ophth Res* 1994;26:65–79.
3. Pastor SA, Singh K, Lee DA, et al. Cyclophotocoagulation; a report by the American Academy of Ophthalmology. *Ophthalmology* 2001;108:2130–2138.
4. Schlote T, Derse M, Rassmann K, et al. Efficacy and safety of contact transscleral diode laser cyclophotocoagulation for advanced glaucoma. *J Glaucoma* 2001;10:294–301.